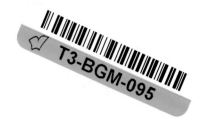

This is my STORY... This is my RHYME

Dr. Sabrina Eileen Mickel

Mickel, Sabrina Eileen.
   This is my story-- this is my rhyme / Sabrina Eileen
Mickel.
   p. cm.
In verse.
ISBN 09779742-1-9

   1. Mickel, Sabrina Eileen. 2. Women dentists--United
States--Biography. 3. Minorities in dentistry--United
States--Biography. 4. Racially mixed people--United
States--Biography. 5. Success--Biography. 6. Family
violence. 7. Courage--Religious aspects--Christianity.
8. Self-realization. 9. Christian biography. I. Title.

RK43.M53A3 2006   617.6'092
                          QBI06-600303

This book is dedicated to the memory of my dear mother,
Mrs. Zelma Glenn

Acknowledgements

You won't believe this, but I did not want to write this book. I did not want to put my life story on paper. However, I believe that the Lord, my God, would not let me be at peace until I did. The thought came to me in 1995 and I started writing but kept stopping and forgetting about it for long periods of time....years. Once my children were born, I completely put this writing aside.

Then, in 2001, the Lord spoke. I felt that He was nudging me to write. He put it on my heart to make this story into a rhyme. This project took over 4 years. As my heart bled for the plight of the majority of African-American children, God made me realize that He wanted me to tell what He has done in my life. So this book is really a testimony. It is particularly meant for children of all races, socioeconomic classes, religions, etc. I'm sure that adults of all ages will also benefit from reading the contents of these pages.

I must acknowledge God first for all the things He has done. I don't even feel as though I made many of the decisions in my life. I believe I was led by the Lord. I know that He kept me. So to God be the glory!

To my dearly departed mother, Zelma Glenn-Burroughs: you encouraged me and my siblings to become anything we wanted to in life. You encouraged us to go to college no matter what. You taught us how to be independent. You were a true jewel. I know God needed you in heaven more than we needed you down here on earth so He took you at such a young age. Thank you, mommy, for all your sacrifices for your children. I can't wait for our reunion in heaven!

My husband, Dr. Andre K. Mickel who I am sure was sent to me by God Almighty: You have encouraged me to do so many things with my life. I love you. You believed in me when everyone else cast me aside. You are my friend as well as my husband. You have a tremendous success story yourself that I know you will put into writing someday as well. You are always supportive and I know that no one, besides the Lord, cares for my total well-being more than you. You are my earthly King. Thank you, Andre. I pray that I am always a good wife and mother "as long as we both shall live".

To my sons, Andre D. and Alexander: I love you both. My heart is yours. I want you to know how hard I worked to give you the lifestyle you are blessed to live. You have far more advantages than your dad and I had at your ages. Please honor us by working hard and making us proud of you. We will be by your side as long as we live. We pray for you continually.

To my mother-in-law, Mrs. Lovie Mickel, who will drop everything to help us with the children or just about anything else! Thank you, mom! Thank you and dad (dearly departed, Archy Mickel) for making my husband the man he is today!

To my mentor, Dr. James Hovell: you gave me a start and encouraged me throughout my entire journey through the road to becoming a dentist. You helped me make the right decisions when there was nobody else I could confide in. You are the BEST role model I've ever had. Thank you, Dr. Hovell.

To my sister, Sophia: I thank God for you everyday. You are truly my friend. To my sisters: Selena, Sophawn and Suzette: I love you all. Thank you for all you do. I pray I am a good role model and I will always be there for each of you until the Lord calls me home.

To my brothers, Milton and Matthew : You are both in my prayers each and everyday. My heart bleeds for you both. I look forward to that day when you return to the Lord with a repentant heart and true commitment to God. He has kept you both through dangers both seen and unseen. There is no doubt about that.

To my brother, Fareed: I found you! With the Lord's help, I found you and I love you. We missed many years together as siblings but God is in control and I know this was His plan. When I was in the midst of writing this book, I wondered when I would end it. I could have gone on and on with my life story. However, when you came into my life, I realized my writing was over. My life has come full-circle. All the years of wonder and doubt about my other biological half had come to an end. Thank you. Thank God for you.

To my friends and church family: there are too many to name but I give special thanks to my friends, Naomi Adams, Shirley Lawrence and the entire Deborah-Ruth Sunday School class, Rev. and Mrs. McMickle for listening and loving me, Martha Jones and Estomarys Tall, who are ALWAYS there to support me. You all are special and dear to my heart. Thank you for every encouraging word and deed.

To my Grandmother, Mrs. Zelma Yancey and all of my aunts, cousins, etc.: Thank you for sharing information that helped me ultimately find my other biological half. May God bless and keep you always.

To my patients: Thank you for supporting me and trusting me to be your dentist. I am truly honored when someone walks into MY office door to be a patient in my practice.

To my Links, Inc. sisters, my Alpha Kappa Alpha sorors, my Northeasterners sisters and my Jack & Jill family: I am honored to be a part of such fine organizations with such rich histories. I hope to use all of my talents to do my part in continuing to make each of these organizations a blessing to ourselves, our families and most importantly, to those less fortunate than ourselves. Remember that "to whom much is given, much is required". God bless you all.

Introduction
By Dr. Andre K. Mickel

She was born to be a great dentist, loving mother, precious wife, caring sister, concerned citizen, passionate Deborah-Ruth Sunday school teacher, skilled seamstress, involved University School parent, dedicated Antioch Baptist Church choir member, best friend, successful business owner, and to me, the most beautiful woman in the world. Additionally, for what it is worth, some call her "soror", some call her "Link sister", some call her Archousa, some call her "Northeasterner sister", some call her Jack and Jill mother, some call her "Alpha Sweetheart", some call her "Boss", and some call her "Ms. President", but for the record, she prefers to be called a "Child of God". Who is she? She is MY wife, Dr. Sabrina Eileen Mickel!

Who could have ever imagined that this little soft-spoken black girl from the impoverished Southside of Youngstown would one day become all of this........and much more by the grace of Almighty God?

Growing up she was often treated as though she was completely invisible by her schoolmates or worse yet, picked on because she was so quiet and not a part of the "In crowd". If they only knew what was going through that fabulously unconquerable mind even as they teased her. "One day I will be a dentist with my own office". Even at a young age, Sabrina somehow knew deep down in her heart that despite people ridiculing the thought that a little girl from the Southside of Youngstown could ever be a dentist ......she was determined to accomplish her goal.

*Interesting Note: Dr. Sabrina Mickel and her husband, Dr. Andre Mickel recently saw one of those ridiculing schoolmates...... as he was bagging their groceries. It did not look like he was laughing then!

I am so thankful today that Sabrina's dearly departed mother, Zelma Glenn had the God given foresight yesterday to ensure the most enriching growing environment and developmental activities that have helped shape MY precious wife. What is even more inspiring is that my mother-in-law, Zelma, was able to accomplish this feat in spite of her severe economic limitations. I never had the pleasure of meeting this great black woman, but wish to dear God that I could tell her how wonderfully thankful I am.

Mrs. Glenn.......The world will now know the inspiring story of your daughter: Dr. Sabrina (Glenn) Mickel! Thank you for MY wife.

To my dear wife....EVEN NOW, YOUR MOTHER IS SMILING DOWN FROM HEAVEN!

This is your story, this is your rhyme.............................

YOUR loving and devoted Husband and fellow Child of God, *Andre*

Forward

By Dr. James R. Hovell

"Life is like a grindstone-either it grinds you down or polishes you." In presenting her life story in rhyme, Dr. Sabrina E. Mickel tells how her dream of becoming a dentist became a reality through hard work, determination, perseverance and dedication. She has become a polished professional, wife and mother because she would not give up her dream.

As a child, her home environment was less than desirable, but with love and encouragement from her mother and a strong belief in God, she was able to maintain her focus and resist the easier route of drop-out and failure.

A mentor is defined as a wise and trusted counselor or teacher. To be a mentor or role model, one needs to be exposed to such an individual. Dr. Mickel's reference to me as that individual who helped her causes me to remember my mentors. Because Drs. James Tate and James Corbett helped make it possible for me to succeed in my dental practice, I have considered it my obligation to help those who have followed me.

In conclusion, I wish to quote one of my heroes, Dr. Benjamin E. Mays, President Emeritus, Morehouse College who states "it must be borne in mind that the tragedy of life does not lie in not reaching your goal; the tragedy lies in having no goal to reach. It is a   disgrace to have no stars to reach for. Not failure, but low aim is a sin".

Dr. Sabrina Mickel reached for the stars as a child and succeeded.

James R. Hovell, D.D.S.

Table of Contents

Chapter 1

A Childhood Misunderstood

I was conceived and born during troubled times.
The struggle for equality was on my mother's mind.
The last position she expected to be in, was toting around a
baby girl then.
Most times the courses our lives take are determined by the
decisions we make.
But in this case, perhaps it was fate that caused my mother to
end up in that state.
She said he took and laid her down.
Then he decided it was okay to boss her around.
Mom said he told her "I'll kill you with this knife...
if you don't let me have my way with you...".
Of course she submitted; what other choice did he give?
Nine months later I was born and I lived.
I never knew the man you would call my father.
Mom said he was Arab, from the Middle East, somewhere.
I'm told that it is a place of unrest, of war and constant fighting.
That's what I've believed even this very moment as I'm writing.

Either way, I'm an American Minority.
I'm female, African-American and Arab; that's my story.
But Hallelujah, it doesn't end there.
I'm also the child of a God who cares!
He keeps me throughout my life when things seem bleak.
My father in heaven makes me strong whenever I am weak.
He is truly an awesome God. To Him be the Glory!
You're about to see proof through my life story.
Read on and pay close attention...
To the many blessings and miracles I just have to mention.

You know they say your life is what you make of it.
If there's something you want, you have to reach out and take it.
My mother constantly reminded me of this fact.
She made me stay focused and remain on track.
She told me I could do whatever I wanted to in life.
She said "You can be a doctor, a lawyer, etc. and still be a wife".
She didn't want my life to turn out like hers did.
When it was all over she had 2 ex-husbands and 7 kids.
Mom dropped out of high school in the 11th grade.
For her, school was not easy and she needed to "get paid".
She went to work in a corner grocery store, I declare!
And that's where she met the man whose blood I share.
Following that fateful day I was conceived, mom had to stop.
She left that store and went to work in a thrift shop.
The boss at the place let her bring me to work each day.
She laid me in clothing bins, put a bottle in my mouth and
started to pray.
She prayed that her life would take a new turn.
That somehow God would smile down on her and then she
would learn
How to make a change for the better and get out of the rut.

It seemed her prayers were answered one day,
when a man named Glenn passed her way.

He came into the thrift store and stared mom down.
"Let's have lunch together someplace downtown".
Mom was flattered. He seemed like a nice enough fellow.
He was wearing a suit and shoes to match in some shade of
yellow.
He impressed her with smooth talk and a charming smile to
match.
Perhaps he was the one; the proverbial "good catch".
Mom told him all about me, the baby she had.
He needed to know that parts of her life had been bad.
He opened up as well and shared his own life story full of things
you'd doubt.
He claimed to have been a survivor of terrible things you only
read about.
It didn't take long before they became a pair.
Mom felt good about this sudden love affair.
Within 6 months they walked down the aisle.
They made me the flower girl and I was all smiles.
What did I know? I was 2 years old back then.
I don't remember the wedding, but I've seen pictures again and
again.

Glenn wanted so badly for this family to work.
He signed the adoption papers and gave me his name.
From that moment on, our lives completely changed.

Chapter 2
Setting My Life's Goal

The years went by and before I knew anything else,
my sister Sophia was on the way. I was no longer by myself.
I didn't know it then, but Sophia would be the closest one.
We fought day and night but we also had a lot of fun.
Then Selena was born, then Sophawn, then Suzette.
Aren't they done having children yet?
Finally along came the boy. Junior was his name.
He was chubby, cute and spoiled just the same.
Now we were a family of eight.
Wasn't that just great?

Life was good, most of the time anyhow.
We were one big happy family, but I wonder now.
There were instances when dad would yell and scream.
He had such a temper. He knew how to be really mean.
I cried when he yelled. I couldn't believe his anger.
But whenever it happened, I felt we were in danger.
A sock on the floor, a spot on a clean dish;

things such as these were enough to send him into a fit.
He spoke with such power and rage in his voice.
It was during those times when I wished mom had made another
choice.
She was very quiet, shy and meek.
She would always tell us how she wanted to "keep the peace".
She said "your dad doesn't need to know everything we do.
He wants to be in control and he's emotionally immature too".

Mom attended church many times each week.
We walked there a lot since it was just up the street.
It was in church that I learned what to do when things went
wrong.
We were taught from the Bible, from praying and singing God's
songs.
Mom wanted all her children to participate fully.
We sang in the choir, attended Sunday school and participated
in plays for Christmas and Easter.
Church was our solace, a peaceful escape
from Dad's rage and anger.
There was only so much we could take.
Mom's extended family attended there too;
our cousins, aunts and uncles and grandma to boot!
That was my life—church, school and family were all that I
knew.
It was enough to make any child "blue".

School was another story I must mention here
Just the very thought of it brings back feelings of fear.
I was the one who stood out in the crowd.
I excelled at many things and made mom proud.
My classmates weren't so happy about my success
Instead they caused me many days of distress.
The girls picked on me and called me names.
The boys were no better, they liked to play games.

I would pretend to be sick as often as I could.
I wanted to leave that rotten school for good!
A girl threatened to cut the ponytails from my hair.
Another girl wanted to coat my hair with Nair®.
I still don't understand why they treated me that way.
I was polite. I smiled a lot and didn't have much to say.
One day my worst enemy, Ericka, confronted me after school.
I still can't believe a girl could be so cruel.
She threatened to beat me because "I thought I was cute".
I stood there in shock, in disbelief and remained mute.
As it happened my Aunt Tara was at my school that day.
She had come to check on her own child to see what the
teacher had to say.
Aunt Tara saw me standing there frightened and upset.
She came over and inquired about why I hadn't already left.
I was afraid to give an answer because enemy Ericka could hear
every word from my mouth.
Aunt Tara got the picture. She told Ericka to leave in a hurry.
She looked at me and said "Sabrina, don't you worry".
She said "I'm tired of hearing about kids bothering you".
"You shouldn't have to be afraid of going to school".
"We're going to put a stop to this nonsense, right now, for
good!"
She told Ericka to leave me alone.
or else she would call her mother by phone.
She would explain how she behaved when the teachers weren't
looking.
Ericka took off running and that terrible day ended.
The next day at school Ericka appeared to be offended.
She made up a story about how tough she was.
She told the other kids a great big lie, just because?
She told them she had kicked my aunt in her pregnant belly
and caused her to lose the baby she carried.
It was all a big lie and an embarrassment too.
Ericka seemed to have a problem relaying what was true.

I think my silence got me into trouble
If only I had spoken up on the double.
I learned a lesson from all that mess.
In spite of it all I am still truly blessed.
The Lord works in mysterious ways, they say.
I see it for myself each and every day.
Just when we think a problem is too big,
God steps in and shows us how small we truly are.
He'll never forsake you and He's never too far.

Mom wanted me to change to a better school that day
So she prayed and prayed that God would make a way.
But there was no money for that kind of a change
Private school tuition was out of our range.
Mom pressed on and checked out school board rules & regula-
tions.
She found out about the "loopholes" in public education.
"A minority student can voluntarily transfer to a majority
district".
Mom's persistent investigation had won us the ticket.
It was God Who revealed that this opportunity was around.
So for junior high school I went to one of the best public
schools in town.
Mom was so pleased to have released me from the torture
Perhaps now there would be some peace in my future.

Meanwhile dad had his own agenda.
He partied with other women "Betty, Jean, Nancy and Belinda".
I believe he loved us but it was difficult for him to show.
He had to play the tough guy, big and macho.
He told me I had to stand up with all my might.
And that I shouldn't always run, sometimes I should fight.
Mom never thought that fighting was sweet.
She reminded me that Jesus said "turn the other cheek".
Mom instilled Christian values in each of her kids.
She said "Give God the glory and indeed you will live!"

Dad didn't go to church with us.
Instead he would make a fuss.
He slept late on Sunday mornings, his bedroom door shut tight.
We had to tiptoe around quietly getting dressed or there'd sure
be a fight.
On weekdays he left early to make it to work by 7 or 8.
Sometimes he worked a double shift. We didn't see him and
thought it was great!
He worked in a steel mill in an adjacent town.
In those days manual labor type employment were the best jobs
around.
Like mom, dad had not graduated from high school.
There weren't many opportunities without that diploma.
He had been in and out of prison for minor offenses.
He told us stories that no one else had witnessed.
There were nights when he said he had no place to lay his head;
so he went to the nearest jail and asked for a bed.
He said the police officers would let him stay there for the night
and actually let him leave in the morning (it just didn't sound
right).
Still dad insisted that he experienced some of the worst situa-
tions that life had to offer.
But regarding this marriage, he was determined to prosper.
His days of living like a bum were over.
He had been on his own since he was a boy.
He had been one of 13 children in a home with no joy.
His mother gave birth to them with the aid of several different
men.
She had never once married but got pregnant again and again.
My dad had fond memories of the man he called "dad".
He had just one picture of him. It seemed very sad.
He told us his father passed away when he was only 3.
Whenever he mentioned his dad, he spoke of him tenderly.
It must have been hard for him living in different places.
He went from home to home, waking up and seeing new faces.

His mother wasn't really concerned. She wasn't really there.
She was too busy having many a different love affair.
When dad married mom, he tried to stay committed.
Surely he wanted a stable environment for his own little nest.
The problem was... he didn't know how since his own family life
had been such a mess.
As mentioned before, he yelled and screamed. That was just his
way.
We literally walked on egg shells each and every day;
always worrying what might "set him off."
His mean streak was enough to scare any child.
His kind side would suddenly appear once in a while.
He could be mad one moment and then suddenly smile.
I suppose his moodiness caused us to fear him.
At any given moment he's happy and nice, then suddenly, angry
and raging.
Many a family picnic or Christmas morning joy
was ruined when he decided to go ballistic and throw around
our new toys.
I recall one Christmas morning my siblings and I were busy
enjoying our new presents.
Then Dad woke up and went into a rage because gift wrap and
boxes were left on the floor.
He came over to me and yelled in my ear that it was my entire
fault that the room looked like a pig's sty.
The next thing I knew he pointed his finger and poked me in the
eye.
I cried and ran to the bathroom mirror. My eye had a bloody
spot.
I couldn't believe he hurt me on Christmas day. Would he ever
stop?
He really knew how to ruin a special day.
I thought many times he must have wanted it that way.
It happened too often to be a coincidence each time.
The very act of ruining your children's joy ought to be a crime.

My mother would say very little when dad went off like a
"kook".
I think she was just as afraid since she remained a bit aloof.
She loved us and prayed daily for our protection.
God must have heard her many cries for help. It was a constant
task.
He always came through once she knelt down and asked.
I could go on and on about daddy Glenn.
But this is my life story. So for now, regarding dad, I'll end.
I said before we were one happy family, or so we thought.
As children we were carefree so the bad things we quickly
forgot.
In the summer, we gardened, grew vegetables and fruit.
We started at 6 A.M. wearing overalls and rubber boots.
We learned how to till ground, how to dig and how to plant
seeds.
To keep our plants healthy we were sure to destroy the weeds.
We played with Barbie dolls, sometimes with the neighbors
across the street.
Our mother took us to the Public Library several times each
week.
We went to garage sales seeking any kind of bargain.
We found household goods, clothing and tools for our garden.
Church was still at the center of everything we would do.
Summer revivals were an annual event we looked forward to.
During the revivals we went to church service every evening for
a week.
After the service, we had good food, fresh lemonade and every
kind of cake.
It made sitting in church every single night well worth the wait.
We had a family picnic for each and every summer holiday.
All of our aunts, uncles and cousins would come to eat and play.
We held our picnics at a park, a beach or someone's backyard.
The grownup's favorite pastime was to challenge one another to
a game of cards.

I thought we were the closest family that God would ever create.
We could count on seeing one another every Sunday. I could hardly wait.
We also had plenty of pets. My first was a cat named Tom.
Tom was so sneaky and jumpy. He always scared my poor mom.
Mom allowed us to ride our bikes as long as we didn't go too far.
If she thought we were gone too long she would come and find us in her car.
She was very, very protective and worried a lot. She was stressed.
She voiced her worst fear many times…. that her children would become victims of sexual molest. As I look back and consider the manner in which I was conceived, mom's fear was easy to believe.
Junior high school was quite a new experience
I had not been around many children from other racial groups prior to it.
The first day was tense for me and mom, for both of us.
My transportation for the first time ever would be the city bus.
On the first day of school mom decided to wait at the bus stop in her car.
She followed the bus to make sure it would actually take me there.
She was so special to have been so protective.
I couldn't appreciate the concern she displayed back then.
However today as I write this I know I was blessed.
God gave me a mother so loving and self-less.
When the bus stopped at the front of the school, the driver looked back at us and said "Cool".
He said "the weather forecast calls for sunshine and warmth".
But all of you on this bus have to get back to the books".
We all let out a moan and headed off the old bumpy bus.
I waved goodbye to mom with a smile but inside I was a mess.
We had to wait outside the school doors until it was time for classes to begin.

I was afraid I would be an outcast again.
In elementary school I had already felt the pain of being rejected.
I was hoping so badly that at this school I'd be accepted.
I looked in front of me and behind me and there were only white faces.
It felt so strange but mom assured me that this would be a better place.
Then suddenly a car pulled up outside those school doors.
A black girl got out and I felt a bit more secure.
I was hoping she'd come and stand next to me.
Instead she went over and stood under a tree.
The school bell rang and everything changed; no longer was skin color on my mind.
All the kids charged forward, their classrooms to find.
The principal greeted us one by one as we walked in the door.
Right away I noticed how special and unique this school was; wall to floor.
The outside was impeccably landscaped with flowers and the trees stood tall.
The inside was immaculately clean; the floors gleaming and all.
The principal was standing at the door with a smile.
He made sure to say good morning to each and every child.
I was worried I'd get lost in those hallways and be ashamed.
We had to change classrooms each time the bell rang.
I also realized as I sat at my desk that my previous school had not prepared me.
Had I not been a quick learner, I may have failed, you see.
I had to learn a lot but I was willing, able and ready.
I wanted to excel and keep my good grades steady.
I put all I had into my schoolwork.
My sisters thought I had gone berserk.
I told my mom how the teachers expected a lot more from each student.
My mom quickly went out of her way to make sure I had what I needed each day.

She went to the thrift shop and found some old school desks.
She set them up in the basement sufficient for me to study the best.
Each day after school she told me to go downstairs
and spend a couple of hours studying alone there.
Meanwhile she was preparing dinner and keeping my sisters out of my way.
Mom was determined to give me every advantage everyday.
She must have just believed that her children could really do it.
And if she stood by us and trusted in God we would all benefit.
She repeated this process with my sisters, Sophia and Selena.
They transferred to the same new school district to follow in my footsteps.

The year was 1978 and suddenly our town was in turmoil.
The steel mills closed their doors and began to lay off workers by the thousands.
My dad lost his job along with many others we knew.
That was the start of our prosperous city turning blue.
Dad was hopeful in the beginning that he'd find a new job.
But time went by and his hope was robbed.
He had been a crane operator. That was his only marketable skill.
It seemed that no other companies needed such a worker, save the long-gone mill.
Dad longed to find a construction company or one that produced steel.
But so did thousands of other dads sent home from that mill.
It was impossible because the economy was changing.
We were entering a new era in our entire nation.
Dad quickly resorted to other ways of "bringing home the bacon".
He started a new business from home, however illegal.
He started off slow but before long his business was "regal".
Suddenly all sorts of people were coming to our home.

The doorbell rang anytime of day without anyone ever first calling by phone.
Mom knew what was going on but what could she do?
She depended on this man for support and her six children too.
Since his source of money was now just a hustle,
It couldn't be put in the bank or there would be trouble.
He didn't give mom enough money for food or bills.
She decided to go to the welfare office and didn't tell.
She received food stamps, a check and felt shame as well.
The next thing I recall is everything falling apart.
Our entire family suffered a broken heart.
But it wasn't unique as many were suffering from the mill shut down.
People were packing up and moving in search of new work in other towns.

By this time I was in the 7th grade and thinking about a career.
One day my school had career day and one speaker was a dentist whose office was near.
I was so fascinated with what he had to say.
I decided I wanted to be a dentist that very day.
He said the biggest bonus was that he owned his own business and that he could not be fired or laid off like the many who worked for the steel mills.
After experiencing what damage lay-offs could do first hand, his words were golden and I wanted to shout and stand.
The dentist told us how he worked with his hands.
He said his job was complicated and difficult but overall it was grand.
I left school that day as happy as I could be.
I rushed home to tell mom all about my new dream.
She told me how my dream could become reality.
She reminded me how dedication and persistence would allow me to become anything!
Mom never said a discouraging word.
Unlike my other family members who felt it absurd

that little Sabrina wanted to become a dentist.
They laughed when they thought of my pulling a tooth.
They felt I wouldn't be strong enough but that wasn't the truth.
Their laughing made me want to be a dentist even more.
There was no doubt in my mind that I could do it. I was absolutely sure!

When it was time to move up to the 10th grade, I didn't follow the kids from my junior high school.
The high school they attended was even further away from my home and that wasn't too cool.
Remember I didn't live in their school district.
I had to get there each day using a bus ticket.
Instead mom allowed me to stay closer to home that was all she could give.
Still, the new school was better-rounded than the one in the district in which we lived.
When I got there I couldn't believe who I saw, my good old enemy Erika from elementary school attended there too.
I wanted to scream and cry. I felt so very blue.
It just seemed unfair that I'd meet up with her again.
She was still mean to me although I wanted to be her friend.
Erika had her "groupies" who would also act very silly.
I never understood Erika's reason for acting like a bully.
She made fun of the fact that my mom was so protective over me.
She tried to make me feel ashamed that my mom hadn't set me "free".
I thank God for mom's protective nature.
Also, I thank the Lord that I was an advanced student and not just average.
I didn't have to share the same classes with Erika and her entourage.
I began high school in honor's classes because of my excellent middle school background.
Again, there weren't many African-American students in the honor's classes to my dismay.

Although throughout the school there was a substantial array.
I made a few acquaintances with all races, black and white.
I wanted to make friends and do what was right.
At the same time I needed to keep my goal of becoming a dentist in mind.
Peer pressure was a burden and honor's students weren't treated very kind.
I recall sitting in church many times reading the book of Psalm when I was worried about the kids at school.
At the time I didn't know that the writer, David had been running from his enemies but I could relate so well to his prayers and his pleas to God. My heart would be so full.

Our home life had taken a turn for the worse.
Home became unbearable for my mom as it was full of stress.
The straw that broke the camel's back appeared on New Year's Eve.
My dad went into a rage over something small. It was hard to believe.
Dad was drunk and wanted mom to go to a New Year's Eve celebration.
But mom had already planned to ring in the new year in sweet adoration;
praising the One who had brought her through the storm.
She felt a strong conviction to go to church that night.
Dad wasn't having it. He put up a big fight.
The word "fight" is an understatement because he really put on an act.
He stomped his feet, raised his voice then he got in the car and left us, in fact.
We were all there in the house as scared as could be.
We had hoped he had left for good or (GOD FORGIVE US) had run his car into a tree.
We really didn't want to see him dead.
But he frightened us so much so that we were afraid to go to bed.

Before long he returned in the same mean mood.
He had decided that mom was going with him by force; he was a hateful dude.
He showed her a gun and told us children to run.
He said "I'll kill your momma. She belongs to me".
We ran to the basement wondering how we would get mom free.
Sophia was the tough one. She wasn't going to back down.
She hid behind the door in close view of the action.
She unplugged the telephone from the kitchen and took it downstairs.
She called "911"; her eyes filled with tears.
Next thing we knew we heard a gunshot.
At that moment we thought we'd hear our mom's body drop.
I think we all must have urinated in our clothes.
We thought he had shot our loving mom who was as sweet as a rose.
We all ran up the stairs as fast as we could.
Dad left through the front door. We thought that he would.
But lo and behold there was our dear mom, standing there crying, her body intact!
I've never had a more relieving moment than that!
She said through the tears that we had to hurry and pack.
We were going to grandma's home never to come back.
You've probably never witnessed 6 children move faster than we did that night.
We packed a few things and in minutes grandma was there to pick us all up.
She was our angel working through God's power to save us from a life of endless torture.
We moved in with grandma for a little while and mom had to file for divorce.
Throughout the whole ordeal mom was as strong as a horse.
We lived with grandma for almost a year.
Those memories I have I hold in my heart very dear.
Grandma was great at healing our sicknesses and sores.

She stood up for us when daddy would come knocking and
threatening to break down her door.
Grandma had a huge St. Bernard dog named "Bandit" who
didn't appreciate dad coming to his home in a rage.
Bandit was our earthly protection from dad's anger as it intensified
day by day.
Today, I thank God for the little things that kept us safe.
I believe that these things happened not by chance alone, but
by God's grace.
The time that we spent living with grandma was an interesting
year.
We were waiting for the judge to separate this family amidst all
the tears.
Mom would sneak back to our house every now and then to get
items we needed and also to get the mail to pay the bills.
She made sure to watch that dad had left before entering in.
The last thing she wanted was to meet up with him by mistake.
My mom was brilliant in the way she handled our "escape".
The divorce was finalized on my 16th birthday of that year.
Dad left the courtroom with a sad face but managed to whisper
"Happy Birthday" in my ear.
It was a bittersweet feeling. I felt like crying.
But it was for the best to keep anyone of us from dying.
We moved back into our own home. The judge said so.
He believed six children and their mother should be there.
Besides, mom had never stopped paying the mortgage and
utilities with the little money she got from welfare.
God is good all the time!
He helps you even when you're down to your last dime.
In times of trouble, He'll be your shelter.
His love, protection and care for you will never falter.

Meanwhile, I started to display the worst behavior of my life.
I started going through adolescent rebellion and caused mom
more strife.

I'm so sorry today. I'd do anything to take it all back.
But what's done is done and there's no way to "back track".
Mom didn't deserve the stress I put her through, you see.
My hormones were raging and boys were interested in me.
The boys pursued me in school and wanted to call me at home.
Mommy said "no calls because studying and homework is what you've got."
I would get mad at her and beg and plead asking "why not"?
She didn't appreciate my words as they were very disrespectful.
She had reared me in "the way a child should go".
So she didn't understand why I was suddenly acting like her foe.
I understand now that many a teenager will rebel.
But mom expected more from me because I had always excelled.
I managed somehow to maintain good grades in spite of my rebellion.
I enjoyed the learning and education in school, but I had few companions.
I believe there's a purpose for everything that has or ever will happen.
People were strategically put in my life to help me go in the right direction.

My first boyfriend helped me stay focused on my school work.
He didn't do it intentionally. My "security" with him kept me from "sowing my wild oats".
My main interest in high school was in education.
I had very little desire for other types of recreation.
My only real past time outside of school was my sewing hobby.
I loved to sew and make my own clothes. A piece of fabric was my canvas.
I could stay up late at night cutting, sewing and ironing to make a new garment.
Before long I was sewing for others. My hobby didn't lie dormant.
I made prom gowns for other girls, matching cummerbunds and bow ties for their dates.

The prices I charged were a real steal for clothing so "elegant and unique".
I'm sure that most of my peers viewed me as a "freak." I wasn't out there trying to be like them. I was more of a "geek".
Plus my mom still took us to church at least four days a week.
I didn't realize it then, but I juggled quite a schedule.
Between studying, sewing, church, the "boyfriend" and family, life was full.
I didn't have time to worry about our state of poverty or why other people were so cruel.
My mother had a hard time with other people as well.
It seemed that she was the brunt of many jokes her acquaintances would tell.
Instead of lending a helping hand in times of trouble, her church members and family members seemed to make her problems double.

Mom applied for and got a job driving a Pre-school bus.
She needed more money to provide for all 6 of us.
Dad never really paid the child support he owed.
Mom knew she had to work herself to help her children grow.
She was determined to change her life for the better.
But old Satan stepped in and started to meddle.
Mom and I met a man one day at a department store.
He quickly zeroed in on us and wanted to get to know us "a bit more".
His first words weren't even very kind. I'll never forget them.
We were standing in the checkout line and he said with a grin,
"You two came all the way out here to buy that thing?" (As if he knew where we lived).
He pointed to the light bulb my mother was holding in her hand.
We both smiled as polite as we were and mom said "Yes" with a giggle.
Her face lit up. I guess she was tickled.

35

Somehow mom and this man engaged in lively conversation.
I was in a hurry to leave that store because it was my Spring
Vacation.
Next thing I knew he gave my mom his telephone number.
I have to admit I was skeptical and hoped in my heart he
wouldn't be a bummer.
Mom talked about this man the whole ride home.
Apparently she liked what she saw. What it was, I'll never know.
That was the beginning of a new chapter in all our lives. We
went through some things that only God helped us survive.
Shortly after that day at the department store, Burney started
coming to our house regularly, knocking on the front door.
He and mom sat at the dining room table talking for hours.
Listening to Burney talk you would have imagined he was a man
of great power, great wealth, skilled and talented. He even
claimed to be a "jack of all trades". (Master of none as they say).
He really impressed my mom and said all the right things.
Within a month of their first meeting, he presented mom with a
little tiny "diamond" ring.
I couldn't believe she accepted. She barely knew this man.
But she explained how she wouldn't get involved any deeper
without his hand.
One day we all piled up in the back seat of Burney's car.
They were going to get married out of town, somewhere quite
far.
We arrived at a little town and stopped at a small courthouse.
There we met with a Justice of the Peace and Burney became
mom's spouse.
We were silent the whole ride home. Our hearts were filled with
strife.
Had this been a mistake? After all it was mom's life.
But in fact we were all affected because he moved into our
house.
Before long he tried to take over and mom remained as quiet as
a mouse.

She believed that wives should submit to their husbands.
Mom read the Bible daily and Burney claimed to be a Christian.
But the rest of the story will reveal that Burney was on a mission.
Many things happened in our home. Some things I'll never
know.
Had mom known any better she would have told Satan to go!
Burney had been married a couple of times before.
He had other children, none for which he provided support.
Bizarre things started happening that no one could comprehend.
Burney began having household "accidents" every now and then.
Once he was in the basement and the power went out.
He started running back up the stairs saying he got shocked.
Apparently he had messed with the electrical wires.
Earlier that same day he had told mom he wished the house
would catch fire.
He said that if the house burned down they could collect
insurance money.
You hear about many scams for easy money, but that one wasn't
funny....
(Just the thought of intentionally burning down a house in
which 6 children lived.)
It was more than a crime. It would be difficult to forgive.
I'm sure that God was protecting us from Burney's evil plans.
You wouldn't believe Burney's plots and all his rotten scams.
The first year of marriage they filed taxes jointly.
But Burney neglected to tell mom that he owed Uncle Sam
already.
So every penny of mom's tax return was taken to set Burney
clear and steady.
I'll never forget how heartbroken my mother was about that.
She had plans for the money and Burney stole it like a rat.
But like a good Christian woman she quickly forgave him and
moved on.
Burney, on the other hand acted as if he had done nothing
wrong.

I would go on and on about Burney because I could.
But I'll be like my mom and keep silent like a good Christian should.

Meanwhile I was still being a rebellious teenager.
I allowed my boyfriend to manipulate me into doing him favors.
My mother was busy working and trying to please her new husband.
So I got away with a lot more mischief.
And as I mentioned before, I'd take it all back if I could.
However, the Lord forgives; resting on His promise, I should.

Chapter 3
College Years

It was time for me to start planning for college.
My plan was to attend immediately as I had always
acknowledged.
The problem was that we had no resources to pay for higher
education.
So again mom prayed and the Lord heard her frustration.
One day mom's cousin Ray informed her of an opportunity.
He said the Army offered college funds for high school juniors
exclusively.
The only thing I had to do was sign up right away.
I had to go to basic training that same summer instead of going
out to play.
For some reason I was all "gung-ho" when mom relayed the
news.
You would think a 17 year old girl would have a different view.
But I was blessed with a mother who supported me all the time.
If she thought I should do something, I tried to do it without
wondering why.

So right away mom called the Army office and they sent a
recruiter.
He sat down at our dining room table and questioned me for-
ever.
He said the whole process was painless and easy.
The first thing I had to do was take a written test which made
me dizzy.
The test was to determine if I had any mechanical sense.
It would also serve to score my I.Q. to some extent.
I then realized that the test only served to place me in a military
job.
I didn't do so well on it. I actually bombed.
I was too worried and nervous if this was the right choice.
Could I make it in the Army with my little girl voice?
My scores were low but they found me a place.
The sergeant signed me up for the medical supply department
with haste.
The next step in the process was a physical exam.
At that point I wasn't sure how much more I could stand.
The sergeant drove me to Cleveland in his own car.
I wondered at the time why I had to go so far.
Once we got there, I was truly amazed, you see.
There were so many young people signing up just like me.
I started to feel better about the entire situation.
Very soon the thought of being a soldier would come to fruition.
Before I knew it, all the recruits were standing in yet another
line.
We were about to take the military oath this time.
It all seemed so formal the way we stood there.
I didn't really know how serious this was nor did I care.
I figured since I was so young and really just a child,
that whatever oath I was taking had to be mild.
I thought that if things didn't go right I'd just quit.
But I was sure I could do this Army thing. I was fit.

Now it was time to return home and go back to school.
I didn't tell anyone I had joined the Army. It wasn't cool.
So I kept it to myself. I had been teased enough.
And I wanted my school mates to think I was tough.
My first experience actually being in the service was unreal.
My mom and I had to drive 2 hours to get to my "weekend drill".
Since I had only joined the Army Reserve my commitment was small.
One weekend a month and 2 weeks each summer was all.
At the drill hall there were people of every different kind.
They were all dressed in camouflage uniforms, wearing combat boots and standing in line.
I came in and stood in the corner, my mother by my side.
Neither mom nor I knew what to do. We wanted just to hide.
A woman came over and asked if she could help us.
I told her I was new and didn't know what to do.
I didn't want to be noticed or have anyone make a fuss.
She said "don't worry about that, you're on your own here yet you won't get anywhere if you just stand here in fear".
She said she would show me where to go and then I felt relieved.
Mom smiled and patted me on the back then returned to the car.
She actually waited for me for 9 hours since we had driven so far.
Those were the kinds of things mom did for me. She even called me "Kitten".
She was there when I needed her and even when I didn't.
Mom literally escorted me everywhere. She even stayed with me at school functions and football or basketball games.
No matter what, no matter when, she was with me just the same.
I was embarrassed about this when my peers were there.
They made fun of the fact that my mom showed so much care.

The time was fast approaching that mom would have to "let me go".
The payoff for her proper rearing would now start to show.
Of course I strayed like many a child.
But thank the Lord my rebellion was mild!

Now back to the first day of weekend drill…..
I watched how most of the soldiers sat around looking for a thrill.
It seemed they had no work to do; no real reason to be there.
The rooms were all filled with donuts and coffee. Each one had their share.
I felt so out of place and worried if what I had done was right.
I didn't even have a uniform. I was the new recruit "on sight".
Each soldier's name was sewn on the uniform's pocket flap.
So I learned many of their names quickly; in a snap!
That first weekend drill ended quickly but I left there feeling funny.
I could hardly believe that for doing absolutely nothing, the Army would give me money.
It was true and the army came through on their word.
The very next week I received a paycheck. It was absurd!
My first paycheck ever! I was so happy I could hardly contain it.
It wasn't much money but right away I saved it.
I still had to finish out my junior year in high school before going away to basic training.

I joined the Army in February so I had four months remaining.
During those 4 months, one weekend each month, I attended Army Drill.
I had to continue wearing civilian clothes and feeling like a misfit until
I could go to basic training where I would receive my camouflage wear.
Unexplainably, I was anxious to look like a real soldier there.

The time passed quickly and my junior year was done.
I left home for the first time to go to boot camp which wasn't much fun.
I cried on the Greyhound bus as I watched my mom drive away.
I thought to myself "I'm officially on my own now." I wanted to stay!
The bus made many stops before arriving at our destination.
From the looks of things we were not picking up people for recreation.
Most of them were young men carrying huge duffel bags.
They too were headed to Cleveland to be shipped out from the MEPS* station.
The bus finally pulled up into the Cleveland terminal.
I had been instructed to look for a military official.
This individual was supposed to transport me to the MEPS* station.
I saw no one who fit that description. Perhaps he was on vacation?
Over in the corner, the "duffel-bag carrying" guys had formed a tribe.
I went over and joined them without saying a word. They too were looking for a ride.
There were men hanging around the bus station watching my every move.
They were trying to be discreet in their staring but they were not smooth.
One man came over to me and asked if I needed a ride.
I said "no, I'm O.K., I'm here with these guys".
Another man approached me and of all things asked if I needed a job.
I can only imagine what he was thinking. I told him "No, I'm with this mob."
The Lord protected me even in the midst of danger.
He put a fence around me to ward off the stranger.
I'll never forget that experience as long as I live.

God was with me. I am absolutely positive.
MEPS- Military Entrance and Processing Station

We then decided to walk to the MEPS station since walking didn't cost.
I'm so thankful that the Lord provided those guys or I would have been lost.
From that moment on I was never alone and didn't need to ask.
In every new situation He provided a buddy to share in the task.
I cannot honestly say that I felt the Lord's presence back then.
It is only now that I realize how faithful He had been.
He was with me day and night to keep me from going astray.
That's why I would be remiss not to give Him the Glory in my story today.
We had to get to the airport once we were processed at the MEPS station.
Again, the military simply left us with a bus ticket to the airport and an airline ticket for the flight to make it all the way to our destination.
This group heading out to the airport was larger than the one before.
Some of us were headed to the same military base but most had no idea what was in store.

By the time I arrived at Fort Dix, New Jersey it was 4 A.M.
I figured they'd let us settle down and nap for a while then.
Little did I know that 4:30 A. M. was "rise and shine time"?
Can you believe we did not sleep? It was a crime!
We were told to go to the Quartermaster to pick up fresh bed sheets.
I was happy because I thought maybe now we would be able to sleep.
To my dismay we were ordered to make up our beds and line back up instead.
We were ordered to go to the "Chow Hall". Were they playing with our heads?

We were not hungry, but sleepy at that point.
I wanted to scream and run from that "joint".
How I wanted my mommy right then and there!
What had I done leaving home at 17 as if I didn't care?
Of course I was on a mission to move up in life.
But I had no idea how difficult the chore would be and full of strife.
Boot camp was tough. The sergeants really did yell and scream.
This experience was for real. It wasn't a dream.
Right away we were taught to march in formation.
We had to be quiet. No one could carry on a conversation.
Fear gripped me as I felt so small.
Thank goodness we were split up into 2 groups, guys and gals.
I was happy we were split because I knew the men were stronger.
If we had to compete with them, our training may have been longer.
The general theme in boot camp was "hurry up and wait".
It seemed we were rushing to our training sites as if we were always late.
The instructors were in no hurry. This was their "9-5".
They were enlisted service persons in no rush to arrive.
We had courses on all sorts of subjects dealing with the military.
We had to pay attention to detail and keep everything absolutely sanitary.
They taught us how to fire weapons and how to identify military rank.
We learned about land mines and even how to identify a foreign tank.
Boot camp was well-rounded. I became a new person during all the hustle and bustle.
I went in weighing 98 lbs. and came out weighing 110-All Muscle!
I'm sure that as you're reading this, you think 110 lbs. is so small.

However, understand that I started at 98 lbs. and 17 years old,
that's all!
Exercise was a major part of each and every day.
Sometimes we would run a few miles. Sometimes we'd stay.
When we stayed by the barracks, we lined up in formation.
We spread out and the torture began... those painful sensations!
We completed one whole hour of jumping jacks and arm and
shoulder rolling.
We dare not quit or we were in for an embarrassing scolding.
The drill sergeant's duty was to yell and scream 2 inches from
your nose.
So I wouldn't dare cry or quit. I maintained the workout pose.
We were told from day #1 that we'd better not play sick.
They also informed us that menstrual cramps were used by
women as a trick.
Of course all the women knew that these men had no clue.
In the case of severe cramps, a woman could be THROUGH!
Nevertheless I hung on. I counted down the days until this
would all be done.
I made some friends there and tried to have fun.
I called home to mom often; fearing something bad might
happen while I was away.
Little did I know mom worried about me just the same and
prayed for me each and everyday?
But again our Lord was there hearing her every plea.
He never failed us. Our constant companion He would be.

The best part of boot camp was what we called "chow".
Since we worked so hard, we were always hungry and ate like
cows!
The "mess halls" were filled with food of all kinds.
It was exciting to line up for meals to see what we'd find.
The sergeants taught us how to eat very fast.
We had fifteen minutes to eat; resulting in "gas".

I remember the hunger I felt everyday I was there.
It was so intense that I would eat anything; I just didn't care.
That must be the reason I gained the 12 pounds in 6 weeks at Fort Dix.
I left that place with a new body; no longer a "stick".

I also recall the duties we were given each day.
I believe the duties served more than one purpose allowing time to pass away.
My least favorite duty was "Fire Drill" at night.
It meant you alone had to stay up while everyone else slept all right.
Literally, we had to sit at a desk in the barracks and stay awake.
Our duty was to make sure that no one tried to enter and no fire started by mistake?
Another "favorite" was mess hall duty. I did it religiously.
My job was to wash gigantic pots and pans; scrubbing and rinsing them tediously.
These pots were heavy and a bit bigger than me.
As I washed them, I had to stand on a step stool to see.
There were many other duties as well, each soldier had her turn.
We were always busy doing something, working and trying to learn.
I recall the first day I was given an M-16 rifle to explore.
I felt a little fear with the rifle in my arms and so unsure.
But before long the entire company was carrying around their weapons effortlessly.
A whole host of very young women armed with rifles; what a sight to see.
The drill sergeants pumped us up about defending the Great USA.
I even wanted to go Airborne. I really got carried away!
Today I couldn't even imagine jumping from an airplane!
I now feel a little fear just getting aboard one. What a change!

I actually thank God for that opportunity today.
It made me a better person; conscious of my ways.
There are many little interesting stories about boot camp that I could share.
But I won't "hog" the story with the details. I'll keep it fair.
There's a lot more to tell about this little life of mine.
The saga continues under my Lord and Savior so Divine.

My graduation day from Boot Camp was exceptionally grand!
Mom and Burney drove up to New Jersey to see it first hand.
Mom was so proud. She couldn't believe how healthy I'd become.
I talked the entire 8 hour ride home to Ohio. They must have been numb.
But they listened patiently to all of my stories and tales.
Little did I know, they had something to share with me as well?
Once we arrived home, my mom revealed the news.
Soon she would be looking for "baby shoes".
I was so angry about my mom having another baby!
I screamed at her loudly, "Are you crazy?"
We can't afford the six kids already in this house.
We barely have enough food to feed a mouse!"
My mother's blood boiled "How dare you get on me!" she said.
"As long as I'm your mother you will show me respect, now go to bed!"
I felt so bad after that incident. I had no right!
Who was I to yell at my mom and make her feel even worse about her plight?
Before long we all accepted the fact that another baby was on the way.
We had enough love in our hearts to welcome this child anyway.
Besides I had to worry about paying for my senior year of high school.
You know the pictures, prom and everything that made it so cool.

I had saved some money from boot camp for this reason.
Now the trick was not to spend it until the appropriate season.
I tried to be very good to my mother and help her out with
money.
A lot of my earnings were used for the rainy days more so than
the few that were sunny.
Burney was not much help to us. He just gave us a hard time.
It seemed his only reason for joining us was to help himself and
pay his fines.
My poor mother was in the same situation as before.
And now with another baby on the way; who could take much
more?
My second brother, Matthew was born on my high school
graduation day.
Mom said Burney did not help her at all along the way.
Instead he whispered in her ear as she delivered….
"I told you not to have this baby anyway". At those words mom
shivered.
What a hateful thing to say when your wife is giving birth!
After that remark how could mom have much self-worth?
Shortly after Matt was born, mom filed for divorce.
It was for the best. She had to get away, of course!
Burney was crazy. He proved it time and time again.
It was pretty clear that he couldn't be trusted as a husband and
friend.
Strange things started to happen that just didn't seem right.
Burney tried to get back at us. It seemed he wanted a fight.
Mom wasn't having it. She just wanted peace.
So we prayed and prayed that it would all cease.
God is so faithful. He put an end to Burney's tricks.
Before I left home for college Burney disappeared.
Mom continued to struggle now with seven kids instead of six.
Fortunately, my entire college education was funded by the
Army and scholarships.

I became one less child to be provided for.
Just as Matthew came into the family, I went out the door.
I attended the Ohio State University since it was not too far away.
If mom ever needed me I could jump in a car or bus and be
home that same day.
It was hard to leave but I knew it was for the best.
I was going off to college to become a dentist.
I felt responsible to help my mom in any way I could.
I realize she had made some bad life choices, but I helped as I
believed I should.
Once I became a dentist, I planned to help her even more.
I had 8 years ahead of me and then I believed I would "even the
score".

Mom drove me to college in the Fall of 1983.
Riding in the car, I watched as leaves fell from every tree.
It made me ponder how my own life was about to change.
I felt weak in the knees and my stomach felt strange.
This was it! I was really leaving home you know.
I tried to fight the tears as they began to flow.
I wondered if I could make it on this big campus all alone.
But I had to be brave. I had to show mom I had guts!
I wanted to make her proud and even help her out of her "rut".
After all, I had survived Army boot camp by myself.
I came out of that in the best of health.
College couldn't possibly be any worse than the military.
Yet fear of the unknown made college seem scary.
Just my luck I had to end up in a dorm room in a high tower.
I was assigned to the 22nd floor. It seemed that the move took
about 7 hours.
I watched as the other students came in with lots and lots of
things.
They had sweaters by the dozens, shoes by the case, foot lockers,
storage carts and so forth and so on.

I wondered who could use all that stuff; it must have weighed a ton.

I had only 2 suitcases packed with all my belongings and earthly possessions.

I didn't have much but what was absolutely necessary to go.

After all, we were going to school to study; not to a fashion show!

Nevertheless, I shrugged my shoulders and moved into the dorm.

I was anxious to see just how this new living situation would take form.

To my surprise, the rooms were extremely small.

Four students were expected to fit into a space the width of a tiny hall.

The bathrooms were shared by 16 student "strangers".

There were 4 commodes, 4 showers, and 4 sinks between us, so I was concerned and the 22nd floor was so high off the ground.

From the room's one tiny window, we could see the whole town.

The campus itself is a city within a city.

I just had to get used to all this and end the self-pity.

Before long, I had the routine down.

I located a school map and found my way around.

My roommates were all different; from many "walks" of life.

I just smiled at them all and tried to be nice.

Many of them implied that they came to college just to have fun.

Some admitted they had to be there or else they'd get "hung".

Most of the freshmen lived in those two tall towers.

It wasn't a pleasant experience, but we had absolutely no power.

Somehow I made it through that first year alive.

It wasn't easy, but well worth the prize.

I remember my first college course examination.

I hadn't really studied. I thought I could just use my imagination.

Just like I did in high school; it was my technique (my trick).

For a test question, I'd sometimes write whatever I wished.

If I couldn't answer a particular question specifically,
I'd expound on something similar to impress my teacher
terrifically.
College was different. "They really expected you to know that
stuff."
The college professors called my "bluff".
Many exams consisted of multiple choice questions.
So either you knew the material or you failed the lesson.
Following that realization, I began to buckle down.
I studied day and night and rarely went out on the town.
I had many college courses like biology, chemistry, physics,
mathematics and psychology. I even had a course in linguistics.
I wanted to do the best I could so I kept on striving.
It was a lot to juggle, between studying and just surviving.
I was very serious about college. It wasn't just something to do.
I had just one chance before all the money would be used.
Some other students partied as often as they could.
I was blessed to have had no desire to "hang out" like they
would.
I kept the goal at the forefront of my mind.
My interactions with others were brief, but kind.
I rarely skipped a class for fear of missing something.
I wouldn't rely on anyone else for information; I mean nothing!
The first year went by quick. In a flash it had ended.
I was fortunate to have made it; for some, college education was
now suspended.
One weekend per month I had to attend Army reserve drill.
Leaving the dorm room in combat attire looking like I was off to
kill.
I was embarrassed for the other students to see me dressed that
way.
Luckily I had to get up and leave the dorm by 6 A.M. on those
days.
I rarely saw anyone so early Saturday and Sunday mornings.
But coming back to the dorm at 5 P.M. was a different story.

I took my books to drill hall to study during down time.
We didn't really do any real work so my studying time was prime.
Other soldiers made fun of my commitment to school work.
They couldn't understand and acted like a bunch of jerks!
I told them that becoming a dentist was my ultimate goal.
They laughed at me and made me feel less than whole.
But again I thank the Lord for guiding me through.
He strengthened me and comforted me in anything I would do.
I met a lot of people at the weekend drill.
These people were from all walks of life; in the Army; for real.
I realize how naive I was as I look back today.
I had become a trained "killer" to get paid in that way.
As long as I was enlisted, there was no threat of war.
And neither had I considered war a possibility anymore.
I would have panicked had one actually come about.
I hadn't understood what it meant to be a soldier, no doubt.
Nevertheless, I pressed on, I had big dreams you see.
No schoolwork, no army, nobody was gonna stop me!
As mentioned before, I barely had enough to get by.
Perhaps I was crazy but determined to try.
Whenever anyone told me "I couldn't", I took it to heart.
Those words were fire in my bones, tearing me apart.
So I took it as a challenge and proceeded to do even more.
The Lord was in front, behind and all around me, I'm sure.
He has a divine plan for everyone's life if only we submit.
We must let His Will be done and never, ever quit.
Those four years of undergraduate studies were moving along fast.
I remained focused on becoming a dentist as each year flew past.
One summer vacation I decided it was time to reach out.
I needed a mentor, a role model, a real live dentist about.
So I looked in the telephone book and found two.
To be perfectly honest I was afraid and unsure of what to do.
I chose two I had heard people in Youngstown mention.
My mission was simple and I had good intentions.

I didn't want anything from them. I'm not a jerk.
I just wanted to see what they did everyday at work.
Afraid to call, I decided to write letters to send by mail.
I requested a chance to see them in practice, every detail.
Also, it was almost time for me to apply to dental school (my
confession).
I wanted to be sure I really understood the dental profession.
Only one of the two dentists responded to me.
He called my home and my mom answered the phone happily.
I went into shock when she requested that I take the phone.
I immediately said "tell him I'm not home".
She looked at me with eyes of stone and blurted out "you'd
better take this phone!"
So I did what my mother told me, especially then.
I said "hello" as I reached for an ink pen.
His name was Dr. Hovell and he was very kind.
He said that if I wanted to observe in his office, he wouldn't
mind.
I had to write down the date and time I would meet him,
I admit.
I was so excited and nervous I didn't want to forget!
Once I hung up the phone my mother said "fine
Now don't you feel better for answering that line?"
I have to admit she was a very smart woman and mother.
My life would have not been the same had I been the daughter
of another.

I remember the first day I stepped into Dr. Hovell's workplace.
I think I had a pleasant smile and look on my face.
I was extremely nervous but didn't want it to show.
It felt very strange being there but I didn't want him to know.
He told his staff to show me around the work space.
They tried to familiarize me but I still felt extremely out of
place.
I was very quiet. I didn't know what to say.
I just watched carefully what he did every single day.

I stood beside him as he saw many patients one right after
another.
I watched him give injections and perform root canals, oh
brother!
I learned a lot about dentistry that particular summer.
It was an enlightening experience and by no means a bummer.
I didn't get paid for standing there 8 hours plus each day.
But the connection I had made and all I had observed was worth
more than any pay.
I had actually made a connection in the dental community.
Now my goal was more set in stone than it was initially.
I was so blessed to have him as a mentor and a friend.
He never discouraged me and never allowed me to bend.
One thing I learned from that experience and opportunity is
that everybody really needs somebody. There is no immunity.

It was time to go back to Ohio State before long.
The summer went by so quickly. I had to stay strong.
The classes got tougher in my junior year just as the time to
apply to dental school drew near.
I hoped to remain at OSU to conserve money.
I still wondered how I would pay, it wasn't funny.
I took on a part-time job to get some cash flow started.
I worked as a direct care aid for the mentally retarded.
Dedicated and determined, I didn't complain nor sob.
I had to work 8 hour shifts at that particular job.
I worked 3 days a week starting at three in the afternoon.
I went to class in the morning and then headed out to work.
It was a hard job as we cared for each beautiful, helpless child.
We would bathe them, feed them, keep them company and our
manner had to be mild.
After working those 8 hours, I'd arrive at my apartment around
11:30 P.M.
I always felt tired, outdone, sweaty and extremely dirty.

So I would take a shower, get in bed, set my alarm for 4:30 A.M.
and curl up.
The alarm rang and up I'd jump, already feeling like I had to
catch up.
I had to study for my classes and do my homework assignments.
It took a lot of motivation to do what I did.
Again, I give God the Glory for only by His Grace could I live.
It wasn't normal to live on 5 hours of sleep each day (especially
when every waking hour you are sweating the day away).
But I was young and had the physical energy and might.
I was never bored nor did I complain about my plight.
I still worried about my mother, brothers and sisters back home.
I wanted so badly to help my family no longer have to "roam".
I wished to be the "savior" to improve everyone's way of life.
However, my goals were unrealistic; much more than I could
"bite".
Still I pressed on with every good intention.
I know now that God was with me. He had a vision.
Until now, I haven't mentioned my love life on purpose.
I'll just say that I had one steady boyfriend on the surface.
Being his girlfriend helped to keep me focused.
I didn't have any desire for more "hocus-pocus".
I was at peace with my so called love affair.
This one "boy" was the only one for whom I cared.
While he was out flirting, partying and having fun,
I was in my apartment studying or at work getting things done.
In my heart and mind I was happy in spite of what he did.
I didn't need him around anyhow acting like a big kid.
I believe this whole ordeal was another way God protected me.
He kept me satisfied with my meager social life- you see.
Sure I had problems with this guy.
There were even times he'd bring tears to my eyes.
Although he ran around with other young ladies;
he was possessive over me to the point of acting crazy.

If I expressed interest in any other guys;
he would blow his top. I'll never understand why.
On one particular afternoon, I was driving and he was the passenger.
I said something he didn't like so he slapped me in the face.
I was behind the wheel of the car!
It was such a disgrace!
I didn't know what had happened at first.
Tears welled from my eyes as I realized I had been struck.
Again, God stepped in and saved me from getting involved in a
potential car crash.
Isn't it awesome how he can come to your aid in a dash?
Had I been smart I would have stayed clear of him.
Instead, I accepted his apology and we "tried" again.
It was only a matter of time before he hit me again.
I suppose it was a way to control me and I could no longer call
him my friend.
I had been hit by my father many times before.
Enough was enough! I had to even the score.
But he put up a big fight as I tried to break it off with him.
He became my stalker; showing up in my territory again and
again.
I just ignored him and finally it all came to an end.
Very soon after that my sister Sophia graduated from high
school and came to OSU.
We lived together for a short time but it was hard to go through.
We had very different personalities and soon the fighting
started.
Unfortunately we didn't last as roommates and eventually
parted.
But Sophia was just as determined as I was to stay and earn her
degree.
She wanted to be an optometrist instead of a dentist like me.
So we went about our own business; each her own way.
We had a much better relationship living separately and it got
better with each new day.

I remember applying to dental school like it was yesterday.
I applied to only 2 schools because Ohio is where I planned to stay.
I really wanted to remain at Ohio State.
And at the same time I didn't want to wait.
I wanted to enter dental school immediately after earning my bachelor's degree.
Becoming a dentist was the only reason I attended college, you see.
Sure, it would be another 4 years of hard work and study.
But whenever I got discouraged, I would call Dr. Hovell, my buddy.
He was a true mentor, someone to look up to, my adopted dad.
Had it not been for his help, things would not have turned out as they had.
I was so blessed as I received early acceptance to OSU!
The college of dentistry was accepting ME!!
I could hardly believe it was true.
For eight years I had waited for this moment in time.
The ladder of success, I was just beginning to climb!
I was so blessed to have had a positive mental attitude.
And for everything I received, I expressed my gratitude.
As any human being, I had my share of issues.
There were many days I used up a whole heck of a lot of tissues.
But somehow God always worked things out.
He kept me many times from having to go without.
It seemed that time went by really fast. It really did flee.
Before long I was graduating with a Bachelor's of Science degree.
I was extremely happy but school was not over yet.
Would I continue with 4 more years of dental school? YOU BET!
After meeting people at the jobs I held throughout my college years,
I realized my best bet was to suffer through dental school and fight the tears.

I saw many people struggling just to pay all of their bills.
Not every employed person was happy, among them alcoholics
and people addicted to pills.
My mom was elated. I was the first to actually attain a degree.
She decided to throw a great big graduation party for me.
She rented a banquet hall and enlisted the help of church and
family.
There was food, a D.J., dancing and fun; all my cousins were
there, each and every one.
Mom displayed my degree and graduation day pictures at the
event.
She wanted everyone to see proof so there'd be no doubt about
exactly how my college years were spent.
It was so beautiful to see how proud my mother was that day.
And in spite of my issues I was glad that I hadn't disappointed
her in any way.

Before long the first day of dental school was drawing near.
Quite naturally, I worried if I'd make it; my heart full of fear.
As I got to know my classmates, I learned they, too were
overwhelmed and nervous.
But we were all determined to learn how to provide dental
service.
Some were becoming dentists and continuing the family legacy.
Others, like me, would be the first dentist in his or her family.
Whatever the case, we were all in this together for the next 4
years.
Not everyone who started would graduate for the #1 enemy was
fear.
Laziness also played a role in the drop-out rate.
Dedication and perseverance would ultimately determine each
student's fate.
We were given a huge box full of instruments and supplies.
I examined each one praying that not one would lead to my
demise.

Our instructors informed us that before long, we'd know how to use each one.

That was an understatement as we spent countless hours using those instruments. I cannot say it was much fun.

As much as I love to work with my hands, dental lab was just too much.

We started out learning the intricate, distinctive anatomy of teeth and such.

We carved whole teeth, root included, from small blocks of wax.

We studied teeth that had been removed from someone's mouth and sterilized in bleach.

I considered these methods of teaching quite unique.

However, we were also given a whole heap load of books, handouts and charts.

We knew we were in trouble right from the start!

Dental lab was just one phase of our training and intense study.

Some studied solo as I preferred to do and others worked with a buddy.

The very first semester we had to prepare for 11 different final exams; what a mess!

I tried not to panic but it was difficult to work out all the stress.

The first two years were designed to prepare us for the last two.

At which time we would turn in our "mannequins" to begin our careers of working on real live people like me and you.

The clinical phase of our training opened a whole new wave of fear.

In spite of the fact we had been preparing for this moment for 2 years, how does one just start administering injections in someone's mouth?

And how does one pick up a drill and start drilling without going too far south?

Sure we had practiced on artificial teeth but now the teeth would have attachments called bodies and brains.

There was no room for error and no one wanted to intentionally inflict pain.

I recall the day we learned to give shots.
I wondered how they would teach us to find the right spot.
Then, to our dismay we found out just how we would learn.
Each student had to pair with another then proceed to take a turn.
We were taught many different types of injections that day.
Each student left there numb all over, in every possible way.
The instructors literally held our hands in order for us to complete it.
Even the biggest, strongest man's hand was shaking. They were having a fit!
And that, my friend, is how a dentist learns how to give shots.
But, of course, there are many other methods in which to be taught.
I'd have to say that day was my most memorable experience of dental school;
(Although there were other events just as "cruel").
I'll spare you all the details of the cadaver dissection since it involved the opening up of human bodies for study and close inspection.
I remember feeling so ill the first day of cadaver lab.
I thought I'd never again be able to eat meat.
To top it all off, Dr. Hovell called that day to take me out to eat.
My favorite food is barbequed ribs and he knew just the place.
But I just couldn't stomach those rib bones staring me in the face.
All I could think of was the smell of formaldehyde.
And all the while my belly grumbled inside.
That aside, I eventually got used to it; cadaver lab became routine.
There was no part of the human body that remained unseen.
I won't continue to give you the whole dental school curriculum.
There's a "state of being" called boredom and I don't want my reader to become a victim.

Chapter 4

Tragedy Strikes

Since this next section was a turning point in my life, I chose to write it in prose in order that the emotions can be more accurately conveyed.

During the beginning of my third year of dental school I was elected president of the Student National Dental Association (SNDA). It wasn't an easy task as I wanted everything to be just right. My first duty as the new president was to plan a trip for our group to go to Washington D.C. for the National Dental Convention. It was July, 1989; a month I shall never forget. To be exact it was Wednesday, July 26, 1989 and the SNDA had a morning meeting. We were finalizing the plans for the trip to D.C. that was to take place that Friday, July 28th. I recall being angry because as president I wanted each of us to represent Ohio State by fitting together like a "well-oiled engine". It seemed that no one else shared my aspirations. Following the meeting, I continued on with my day attending the afternoon classes. All of a sudden my sister, Sophia walked into the clinic classroom. She said she had something important to tell me but that she'd wait until the class ended.

I knew it had to be serious for her to come to the dental school to find me. I excused myself to speak with her. She proceeded to tell me that our grandmother had called and said that our mom was in the hospital and we needed to come home right then and there.

I got a lump in my throat and a dry mouth at the sound of those words. We rushed out of the school and I called my grandmother. She wouldn't tell me anything other than "come home now".

Hurried and worried, Sophia and I packed a few things in a bag and took off for Youngstown in my car. We speculated the entire trip home about what could have happened to her. We cried a little and shared stories about other people we knew who had ill parents. We figured she must have had a heart attack and was hospitalized. She did have hypertension and was on medication for it. Just a few weeks prior to this she had gone to the emergency room complaining of severe headaches and was told she simply had sinus problems. I had just spoken to her on the phone the night before and she said she had been feeling a lot better. The headaches were gone and she was happy. She finally felt good about her life. She had recently earned her GED (General Education Degree) and was taking college courses to earn a degree in early childhood education.

We tried to figure out why she had become severely ill at such a happy, productive time in her life.

As we approached our home in Youngstown we saw many cars parked on the street and people sitting on the front porch. It was a sunny July afternoon. Upon seeing all the relatives and friends at the house, I knew the news couldn't possibly be good. I ran out the car and asked my Aunt Tara "How is she?" Tara took me into the house away from everybody else and I immediately knew my dear mother was gone. I said "No Tara, no, no, no, no,no,no,no!' She hadn't said a word. She just held me and tried to comfort me but I couldn't believe what was happening. "What happened, what happened?" I repeated over and over again. She responded that they didn't know. All she knew was my mom (her big sister) had collapsed while in class at Youngstown State University and was pronounced dead when the ambulance arrived. The paramedics tried to revive her, but to no avail. My mom had passed away at the age of 46! Tara said the coroner would be calling me the following day after the autopsy to tell us the cause of death. I looked around the room and saw all my brothers and sisters and wondered how we would make it without our mother. There were 4 minor children left without parents. Sure, Glenn was still alive and so was Burney but neither man would take the responsibility. Grief-stricken and feeling completely helpless, I allowed my aunts and grandma to make all the decisions from that point on; from funeral arrangements to what would now happen to my younger brothers and sisters. But there was one catch, no one offered any money to help pay for the final expenses.

One of the first calls I made through the tears was to Glenn's mother. She was so mean! I was calling to ask if she knew how I could get in touch with my dad. I said "Hello grandma, this is Sabrina, Milton's daughter". She immediately cut me off and started yelling and screaming, "You better call him your daddy! I don't care what happened between him and your momma, he is still your daddy!" I cried even harder. She made me feel so bad and so frightened that I could hardly speak. Somehow I managed to mumble out the words "my mom died today". The next thing I know she was screaming out "Oh Lord, Oh Lord, No ,No!" Then she finally said she would call my dad and tell him to contact us. She kept saying "I'm so sorry". I hung up the phone. My feelings were hurt and my spirit was completely broken. I didn't care to eat or sleep.

My mother's sisters and cousins had flocked to our house. I was under the impression that they were going to help pay for funeral costs and burial and whatever other expenses there were. I was wrong. Nobody offered. In fact I was told to call the welfare office and ask what they provided for the death of someone on welfare. I made that call but I could hardly talk to that person because of how heart-broken and tearful I was. The amount they provided was so insignificant that I decided it just wasn't worth it. So I called my friend Dr. Hovell. He was so wonderful! He even postponed going to the dental convention in Washington D.C. to be with me and my family.

His father-in-law owned a funeral home in town and he helped us get the best price on the purchase of a casket and provided what we needed to have a funeral right there at the funeral home. I used credit cards. I had used credit all throughout college to make ends meet. As I said before, the Lord puts people in your life at certain times for a reason. His way is Divine. "He is able to do exceeding and abundantly more than we could ever ask or think" (See Ephesians 3:20)*. Dr. Hovell even provided 7 roses from his own garden for each of my sisters and brothers and I to place in the casket on the day of the funeral. Dr. Hovell helped to make it all more bearable.

I have to admit that immediately following the death of my mother, I began to doubt God. My faith wasn't yet strong enough. I wondered like many who have lost loved ones so unexpectedly, "How could God let this happen?" Where was God when my mother was dying?

The coroner called me the day following her death and told me that she had suffered a fatal cerebral aneurysm. He said there was no chance for survival whenever that particular blood vessel completely bursts in the brain as had happened to my mom. I became angry. I asked the coroner if her recent headaches could have been a warning signal. I also asked if an aneurysm could be detected ahead of time before it ended this way. He answered "yes" to both questions. He said that sometimes a CAT scan can detect the weak vessel and the severe headaches could have been a result of the vessel bleeding internally. I immediately thought of mom's recent visit to the emergency room. I became enraged that the doctor had not performed a CAT scan for my mom! She had appeared at the ER at 6:00 A.M. in severe agony. She even had grandma drive her there and the doctor just dismissed it as sinus pain. Who shows up at the ER FOR THE FIRST TIME IN THEIR LIFE at 6A.M. complaining of a severe headache at the base of their skull and the diagnosis is simply sinus congestion? And to top it all off it was July, the hottest month of the year! I also went to visit my mom's primary care physician. I needed some answers. I asked him what happened since he had been treating mom for so long and recently gave her medication for the headaches and she had been under his care for hypertension for many years as well. His response was "things like this happen". He told me that his mother-in-law died the same way. I asked him at what age his mother-in-law died. He responded that she was 82! I walked out of his office furious! My mom was only 46!

I told my grandmother that I had to file a lawsuit. She was against it. She said that it isn't right to sue a doctor. I didn't agree under the circumstances. Here I was in school to earn the title "doctor" and my instructors insisted on excellence. When we were unsure of anything we had to rule out every possible diagnosis before coming to a conclusion about a final diagnosis. I felt I just couldn't let this doctor off the hook that easily. My mom was dead! I'd never get to see her again or talk to her or hug her or tell her that I love her ever again! It was too much to bear! Also SHE was in college; trying to move up in life. She was just beginning to climb the ladder of success herself! It all seemed so unfair. I was angry with both God and the doctors! Who would feed my brothers and sisters? Where would they live now that mom was gone?

Grandma and my aunts decided for us that grandma would move into mom's house and take her place as their care-giver. My thought was that Sophia and I would take them to Columbus and we would rent a big house and just make the best of the situation while remaining in college. I was only 2 years from becoming a doctor. Mom would have never agreed to my leaving school. But grandma actually wanted to move in and make that sacrifice. So that's how it happened. We were very grateful to her for what she did and I told her that as soon as I graduate, I would take the kids to live with me. I also told her that I would help in any way I could and I did just that!

Back to my rhyme

As hard as it was, life had to go on.
I constantly worried about Milton, Matt, Suzie and Sophawn (so-fawn).
My classmates were so kind. They had taken up a collection.
Instead of flowers, they sent money, a more practical selection.
I cried on a whim. It didn't take very much (someone saying "I'm sorry"; a sympathetic look and such).
My instructors were also kind. They helped me catch back up.

I felt such a void in my life I tried to fill it by getting a new little pup!
I "adopted" a 2 pound Chihuahua and named her "Chica".
I took her everywhere with me and nicknamed her "Chica Pica".
She accompanied me to the dental lab after hours.
Even at 2 pounds she liked to exert her little power.
She barked at the other students who were there working as well.
I tried to keep her in my pocket but she wanted to play as anyone could tell.
School was changing everyday we were there.
We were given less bookwork now to concentrate more on patient care.

After all we were training to be dentists.
Working with real patients would be our "life sentence".
Fortunately, I was blessed with good hand skills.
But I had to practice to get even better still.
I recall the first patient I ever saw for a filling.
I thought my hand would shake while "drilling".
Instead, everything went well.
The dental instructor was pleased; I could tell.
He said "you are a natural, a smooth operator, a star. Keep up
the good work and you're sure to go far."
I left the clinic feeling mighty good that particular day.
My ego had been stroked in a most positive way.
But I didn't want to get above myself and have my head "swell".
I was sure that if I let that happen I would lose and fail.
There was a whole lot yet to be learned.
Furthermore, there was a degree I still hadn't earned.
We were required to do this and expected to do that.
There was so much to juggle I felt like an acrobat.
All of it was necessary preparation for the future.
Besides "drilling and filling" we learned extractions and how to
suture.
We had to make crowns, partial and complete dentures.
Dental school was challenging. It was truly an adventure.
I tried to stay active in the Student Dental Association.
But with all I had been through and all the work ahead I was
only concerned with graduation.
One day the student association went to Cleveland for a
seminar on diversity.
We met other students from Case Western Reserve University.
There were about 6 other minority students from Case.
Among them was a young man who made my heart race.
I ignored him so as not to show my emotions.
We talked briefly that day face to face.
And discovered we were from the same place.

When the seminar ended, the Ohio Staters and I headed back
southwest.
I filed his memory away in my mind and wished him the best.

Chapter 5

Finally.........Dr. Sabrina!

Those last two years of dental school went fast.
I had become a dentist at last!
I knew my mother was smiling down from heaven above.
Although she couldn't be there, I still felt her love.
When a mother's child earns the title "Doctor", oh what pride
and joy!
Even more special was the fact that I'm a girl, not a boy!
Mom's famous words to me were "Brina, You can become
anything".
It was a bittersweet feeling of accomplishment having heeded
her uttering.
I knew it was the Lord who guided me through.
It is always necessary to give credit to Whom it is due!

The graduation ceremony was special in every way.
Even my dentist friend and mentor came up for the day.
As I walked across the stage with my degree in hand,

Dr. Hovell came up and handed me a small box closed with a
rubber band.
My classmates surrounded me as I took my seat.
They were as curious as I to see the special treat.
There were 500 business cards in a little case.
Each card read "Dr. Sabrina Glenn" in the same space.
He had created these special business cards for me.
I was as thankful and as pleased as I could ever be.
There was a pink rose on each card next to my name.
My "new" business address and his were one and the same.
Dr. Hovell treated me so special; I felt I owed him a lot.
He was very generous to me; selfish he was not!
So that was the start of a whole new life for me.
No turning back now. My future was set you see.
I was a doctor now, so all my problems had ended, honey!
But I had a small problem, where was all the money?
Apparently someone had left out a few important facts;
although I had stayed on the right track.
Well, I went to work in Dr. Hovell's office part-time;
trying very hard just to make a dime.
At Dr. Hovell's urging I put in a year of hospital training.
More lectures, more instructors, more work, more straining.
To me it seemed like a waste of time because I was broke!
I was paid a small salary, but it went up in smoke.
However, there was a surprise waiting for me, I declare!
The young man I had met two years earlier was there!
I suppose he wanted this hospital training as well.
So we spent the next year together and it was swell.

Chapter 6
My Husband, Dr. Andre Mickel

In the beginning I thought little of this Dr. Andre Mickel.
He seemed so arrogant and self-confident, it gave me a tickle!
We had our disagreements over things both big and small.
But he always dressed the best, so handsome and tall.
We were 2 of a total of 6 dentists working there.
Andre and I were the only African-Americans, but we didn't care.
After all, we were used to being in the minority.
However, Andre took over as though he had seniority.
I admired his self-control and his ability to lead.
Things didn't bother him, even the most evil deed.
How I wished that quality would grace me.
Perhaps then I could be set "free".
Anyhow it didn't happen and I remained the same.
Then one day something happened that caused me to feel ashamed.
One of the other dentists shared with me what was said behind closed doors.

It seemed that our director had some racial insecurities and
what's more;
He made" off-color" comments about Andre and me.
He said he didn't think 2 blacks should be in the clinic together,
you see.

At first I got a kick out of it and took it as a joke.
But when I mentioned it to Dr. Hovell, his anger was provoked.
I panicked as the sweat ran down my brow.
And I couldn't take the words back now;
although I desperately wanted to make it all end.
Something was happening right there and right then.
Dr. Hovell said he planned to call Dr. Baker first thing in the
morning; what a mess!
Dr. Baker was the hospital administrator. Now I was stressed.
This whole thing was blown out of proportion I thought.
But there was nothing more I could do. I was caught!
Immediately I called Andre to get his thoughts on the matter.
He was surprised by my call and even a bit flattered.
He told me not to worry; but I couldn't help my anxiety and
fear.
I felt that because I told a major "war" was near.
It moved me to uncontrollable tears.
Still I felt some reassurance just by talking about it all right.
I saw a completely different side of Andre that night.
He calmed me and made everything seem all right.
I really felt that he was on my side and would help through this
plight.
So that was the start of true love brewing in my heart.
After all the times I hadn't been so nice to him, he still cared
about me even from the start.
Well it all happened in October of that year.
One thing led to another and soon Andre and I called one
another "Dear".

The incident with our director was quickly resolved.
He apologized to us and the problem was solved.
Little did he know that because of all this mess,
Andre and I had truly been blessed.
We were now together as our relationship grew stronger by the day.
We helped one another in many kinds of ways.
There's something else I must mention here.
I still had another man in Columbus calling me "dear".
His name was Tim and we had dated a while.
But something was missing between us. Our relationship was foul.
Still I had trouble telling Tim that my feelings had undergone a change.
The whole situation felt totally strange.
He would still come to Youngstown to visit me.
But I had a burning desire to say "Tim, Flee!"
Finally I got up the nerve to tell him that I had fallen in love.
And I truly believed that my true love was sent from up above.
He was of course shocked when he realized I was talking about someone else.
I felt so bad for him and never intended to hurt him nor myself.
However, the following weekend, Tim decided to surprise me and take a stand!
He showed up at my apartment; engagement ring in hand.
I couldn't believe it. He was trying to propose, but why now?
He tried to make a commitment but didn't exactly know how.
Since it's best to do that before your girlfriend leaves you!
Still I felt so bad for him that it actually made me feel blue.
Wouldn't you know I accepted the ring that day?
I told him I needed to think it over. I needed to pray.
After all I cared about Tim. We had dated for 3 years.
Still all I could do was wallow in my tears.
I was torn because with Andre I felt alive. He was my king!

On the other hand I felt I owed Tim something.
But was that "something" my hand in marriage for my entire life?
Did Tim really want to have me as his wife?
I went back and forth for weeks on end.
I thought I had it figured out every now and then.
But as soon as I made up my mind about one, the other would do or say something to make it come undone.
I recall thinking I just needed to stay with Tim.
After all, we had been together and I really knew him.
Then one day something happened that I shall never forget.
As I thought about Andre, I felt my heart actually "tick".
It ticked so hard I had to go somewhere and sit.
It also felt like someone was pulling down on it.
At that moment I knew God was speaking to me.
He stopped me from blocking my blessing, you see.
God intended for Andre and I to be a pair.
He worked through my heart to make me aware.
I listened because the feeling was so very strong.
I knew then and there that marrying Tim was wrong.
Tim was hurt but he soon moved on with his life.
Then, on Christmas Eve, I accepted the proposal to become Andre's wife.
Just about everyone we knew was shocked and surprised.
The fact that we got engaged so soon was analyzed.
Meanwhile I was in "7th heaven" dreaming of my wedding.
But all the work, I was dreading.
I rallied up support from my aunts and cousins who lived near.
They had all the resources so I had nothing to fear.
They knew a wedding coordinator, a pianist, a photographer and a D.J.
A videographer and a singer; soon my wedding was underway.
Andre went with me to pick out my wedding gown.
I was so excited that I accepted the first one we took down.
Once I tried it on, I felt so beautiful, my image I admired.

I had never seen myself in such gorgeous attire.
Andre saw me in the dress although it was unconventional.
They say the groom shouldn't see his bride's dress, but it was
unintentional.
One thing we had in common was a disregard for superstition.
I wanted Andre to see and like my gown on his own admission.
I had enough sisters, brothers and cousins for an all-family
wedding party.
This wedding was going to be a big event. We were gonna
"party-hearty"!
I put my creative side to work in order to save money.
Andre and I were going to "foot" the entire bill (not funny).
So I made (sewed) 2 of the 4 bridesmaid's gowns and my aunt
Margie made the other 2.
I even made all the flower bouquets. It seemed my work would
never be through.
In spite of it all, I refused to be defeated.
And the anticipation grew as each task was completed.

Let me take a moment to witness to God's wonderment.
The fact that Andre and I had come together was no accident.
As it turned out Andre ended up doing the hospital residency
where we fell in love "by default".
He had previously applied for a dental specialty program in
Endodontics but got no immediate response.
But when he applied to the hospital program he was accepted
right away.
However, following the signing of the hospital contract, the
Endodontics Program called later that same day.
Quite naturally, his first choice was to remain in Cleveland and
get started on his post-doctoral training.
He didn't want to turn down an opportunity like this especially
since the competition was so stiff.
But he was stuck in the 1 year contract with the hospital.
It wasn't time for him to become a specialist at all.

So he prayed and God granted him an edge.
The Endodontic director gave him an unusual privilege.
He was able to sign a contract for the following year.
And he was told "this is the first time we have ever done this
here."
Wow! What an amazing testimony of God's grace.
How he can make a way out of no way as we run this race!
To this very day Andre believes that God sent him to
Youngstown that year just so that he could meet and marry me,
"his dear".

The wedding arrangements were coming along just fine.
Andre's mom and dad offered to pay for our honeymoon "in the
sunshine".
Mom said "pick any place you'd like to go on us".
My dream had always been a honeymoon in St. Thomas.
My fiancée agreed and the arrangements were set.
I wanted to go right then and there but we weren't married yet.
Finally the wedding day came and I was a mess.
I wanted everything to be perfect, from the ceremony itself right
down to my dress.
I made all my brothers and sisters get up early that day.
I wanted no excuses. Everything had to be beautiful and special
in every way.
The limousine drove us to the church in a twinkle.
We all got dressed at the church so our clothes wouldn't
wrinkle.
Earlier that day we had all gone to the banquet hall.
We decorated it ourselves. My sister, Sophawn did the best work
of all.
She made a very stunning centerpiece for the head table.
In the area of creating and decorating she is extremely able.
It all came together so well and so fast.
The hall was ready for our 300 guests at last.
It rained very hard on my wedding day.

Ohio's weather is so unpredictable in May.
I wasn't happy about the rain. It was so gloomy and dark.
That meant we couldn't take pictures at the park.
But lo and behold, my fiancée had another plan.
He called the Art Museum and made his case to the man.
He said,"Today is my wedding day and I really need your help
right now."
It's raining outside and we need to take pictures somehow.
He asked, "Can we come there after the wedding to take pic-
tures in your beautiful marble staircase setting?"
At first the man resisted but Andre said he would make it worth
his while.
So the man agreed and we had a beautiful place to take our
wedding pictures. We were "all smiles".
The wedding took place exactly at 1:00 P.M. at my mother-in-
law's insistence.
She said we would not make our guests wait although there
would be resistance.
It was a beautiful ceremony and beautiful people were attending.
I became more nervous each time I looked into the chapel and
saw it filling.
My sisters all looked so lovely, each wearing a black and white
gown.
They carried pink rose bouquets laced with white ribbons as
they marched down.
The music was so sweet and romantic. Pink and white flowers
and candles graced the aisle.
The voices of the singers were perfectly resonating throughout
the church all the while.
My two cousins had just rolled out the white plastic runner for
me.
The flower girl then sprinkled it with rose petals . What a cutie!
I grabbed daddy Glenn's arm as we headed down the aisle.
Although my heart was racing, I still managed to smile.

As I walked, I noticed my heels were getting stuck.
They were piercing the plastic runner. It made my walking extremely tough.
I must have appeared to be marching and stepping high;
smiling and waving at the guests as I walked by.
The aisle seemed so long that it might never end.
I watched everyone's expressions; lots of smiles and grins.
Andre was already at the altar waiting for me, his bride-to-be.
The closer I got to him, the less I felt anxiety.
He gave me strength and made me feel free,
(And to think that we were about to become family).
I believe the ceremony was beautiful, short and sweet.
Although we said traditional vows, the pastor gave the audience a "treat".
He boldly asked Andre, "Would you be willing to die for your new wife?"
Andre replied, "Yes, she's worth my life."
I must say I was both surprised and taken aback.
Had he replied "No", it would have been a tense moment.
In fact......
It was an awkward question to ask of the groom.
Especially in front of everyone before "jumping the broom".
Thanks be to God that it all went so well.
Our families were pleased as anyone could tell.
At some point during the ceremony, emotions ran high.
As I looked around at the wedding party, there was not one dry eye.
My brothers and sisters were all in tears.
Tears of joy, I hoped and not tears of fear.

When the ceremony ended we piled in the limo car.
First stop was the museum for pictures. I felt like a star!
Then it was off to the reception hall for our big celebration.
We had tons of food, beverages and cake. Everyone was ready for recreation.

The party was grand and we all had fun; from the eldest
individual to the youngest child; each and everyone!
I was exhausted although the day went fast.
Both Andre and I felt relieved when it ended at last!
We had pulled it off but it seemed too good to be true;
A big wedding on a tight budget and a honeymoon too!
We received some nice gifts and lots of cards containing a total
of $1000 in cash.
Andre felt we should take all of it on our honeymoon, the entire
stash.
I said, "Oh no, we only need about $100 for the entire trip".
Andre laughed at me saying, "$100 won't even cover the tips."
It was then that I realized my life was really taking a new turn.
The poor little girl from Youngstown still had a lot to learn.
We thoroughly enjoyed our plane flight to "paradise, in love".
We were as happy and as carefree as a pair of doves.
We landed on the island of St. Thomas in the late afternoon.
Our first night was spent having dinner on the beach in perfect
view of the moon.
In the darkness we heard the waves crashing ashore.
I adored the cool, sandy beach and couldn't wait to see more.
We settled down for the night cuddled up together.
What a peaceful escape. I felt as light as a feather.
I awoke the next morning to the sound of a loud horn.
It took my breath away; a cruise ship was sea born!
I awakened my husband as I kept yelling "WOW"!
"Andre let's go out there. I must see it right now!'
I can't describe the feeling; it was so intense.
I was overjoyed, elated, thankful to God and holding Him in
high reverence.
What a mighty God to have created such beauty galore!
I'd never seen anything this breathtakingly beautiful in my life
before!
Both the sea and the sky were boldly blue.
The tropical feeling enveloped me. It was all so new.

I could go on and on forever about this.
I recall wishing my brothers and sisters could experience St.
Thomas.
But I was on my honeymoon; meant for just two.
Still I wanted my other loved ones to share in it too.
We had a great time but it ended too soon I believe.
It wasn't long before we were packing to leave.

Chapter 7

Moving and Starting My Own Dental Practice

Back at home we had just a month to go before the hospital
program would come to an end.
With all the preparation for our move to Cleveland, we had to
contend.
Andre had to begin his endodontic residency July the first.
Trying to find a suitable apartment was the worst!
Andre did not want to be too far from the dental school.
He wanted to be close enough to walk. He's no fool!
Neither of us had a very reliable car at the time.
Andre had an old Chevy Chevette. I had a VW lemon (or
lime).
He took his education very seriously as I soon discovered.
The work load was so intense I thought he would be smothered.
But Dr. Andre Mickel put his heart and mind into the course of
study there.

He had very little time with me and, at first, it didn't seem fair.
Plus I had difficulty adjusting and did not have a job.
Within a couple of weeks, I felt like a useless slob!
I was looking to associate with a dentist as I had done with Dr. Hovell before.
The task turned out to be more of a challenge than I was ready for.
It just so happens that Andre's uncle owns a dental supply company and knew many dentists in the city.
He took me to meet them and see their offices to alleviate my self-pity.
I had hoped that perhaps one of them would offer me a position.
But no one mentioned it to me; not one clinician.
I did end up with a couple interviews from ads I had responded to.
However, neither dentist called me back. I guess I was just "too new".
One dentist asked me to come in for a "try-out" day.
I treated some of his patients without pay.
He said I had done a great job and he was impressed.
I thought he would call me and offer me a job; I confess.
Instead I kept calling his office and getting the same response like a "tease".
"He's with a patient. May I take a message, please?"
Then one day after a couple weeks, he called me around three.
He said he had hired another dentist but not me.
My smile immediately turned into a frown.
Tears welled up in my eyes. I was so angry with that clown!
I had waited two weeks for his call.
I hadn't done any job searching during that time at all.
He led me to believe that he was getting a job contract together for me.
But as it turned out, he had other plans, you see.
Within a few days I forgot about the clown.
I resumed my job search all over town.

Finally, I came across a dentist who hired me on the spot!
He spoke positively about my joining his practice.
However, he acted like a "big-shot!"
He bragged about all his patients and how much money he made.
I was immediately "sucked-in" because again, I desperately needed to "get paid".
So I started work at his office the very next morning.
He procrastinated about drawing up a work contract and that should have been my first warning.
To my dismay, there were not nearly enough patients for me.
And our verbal agreement was that I'd receive 30 % of the patient's fee.
Unfortunately, I saw only one or perhaps two patients each day.
It just didn't add up to any reasonable amount of pay.
This went on for approximately two months. Then my patience was "shot".
Andre said "We'll get you your own practice in an ideal spot".
I laughed at the idea thinking it to be an impossible dream.
But Andre was serious. He actually held me in high esteem.
So we started making plans and provisions.
I was both excited and scared at the vision.
"Little me"- a business owner? It was hard to conceive.
But before long we had a plan that we could both perceive.
I remember long nights sitting up "putting figures together" on paper tablets.
Andre would chuckle when I read the things aloud that I had written down. It became a habit.
I was trying to figure out how many patients I needed to make "X" amount of dollars.
I tried to figure out financial risks and rewards like I was some kind of a mathematical scholar.
The many pages I had written were my blanket of security.
I needed reassurance that this business could reach maturity.

Fortunately, I had maintained a good credit rating throughout
my career.
I had used credit cards and loans to help make ends meet during
my college years.
My credit rating made it easier to be approved for a business loan.
Much of the application process was completed by phone.
I did, however, run into some "red tape".
The bank requested that if my husband cosign, then I'd be in
ship-shape.
So after a long discussion, we agreed to the terms.
I received my first $100,000 dollars, firm!
It seemed like a fortune as I wrote; nervously signing the promis-
sory note.
Andre's uncle, Eugene was instrumental in getting my office set up.
He had done it many times before so we relied on his experience
instead of a "toss-up".
I had completely cut off my relationship with the dentist in
whose office I would "sit".
He said he'd be mad at me if I quit.
As I saw it, I had no other choice. It was a disgrace so I asked
him why he had hired me in the first place.
His response was "when you walked in the door, you were what I
was looking for".
Then I realized his intentions had not been proper.
He was going through a divorce and had admitted to being a
"bed-hopper".
I thank God that he saved me from all that man's mess.
He was wasting my time and giving me stress.
God had another plan for me.
He wasn't going to allow me to suffer forever, you see.

My plans were coming along for the new business venture.
I found an office building with a suite for rent. It turned out to
be an adventure.

I called the manager and inquired about the building suite.
I thought I was calling the medical building and the manager
informed me that it was across the street.
He asked, "Were you hoping to get into a medical space?"
I said "Yes", but anyhow I can come and see your place."
"Your advertisement sounds like what I am looking for".
The price was right and it was in the area I wanted to explore.
So I went to the building accompanied by Uncle Eugene.
His presenting "me" as the dentist must have been quite a scene.
The manager politely welcomed us and explained every detail.
However, he must have figured that my business would fail.
Just like the bank, he asked if my husband could also sign the
rental agreement.
This time I decided to fight back in utter disagreement!
I responded with this question, "Do you also ask wives to cosign
for their husbands?" "All of them?"
At first he didn't quite understand so I clarified it for him.
"If my husband were standing here in my place desiring to rent a
space from you, would you ask him to go home and have his
wife sign the lease too?"
The manager answered "no" to that question and actually
apologized for thinking unfairly!
At that point I knew I had found the right place to set up my
new practice squarely!
It took several months to get the office together.
We started in the winter so the contractors tried to blame the
weather.
I knew better because they were working indoors for this.
They were converting a lawyer's suite into a dental office.
I had to buy thousands of dollars worth of equipment and
supplies.
It added up to over the $100,000, to my surprise!
Somehow I didn't worry if it would all work out.
My faith helped to melt the clouds of doubt.
I also got a job at a dental clinic part-time…3 days.

I figured I could supplement my income that way.
While the office was being built and furnished, I worked at that clinic unafraid.
And every now and then I came over to see the progress the workers had made.
They promised my office would be ready to move into by March the 8th.
I was banking on it as the bills had to be paid without delay.
Of course they didn't meet their deadline and I began to panic.
I wondered if I could even stand it.
But I had to wait as I had no other choice.
It didn't matter if I raised my voice.
Soon time went by and a new problem surfaced.
Now I had to figure out how to get patients in my door.
As soon as my office phone was connected, I checked for messages every hour (maybe more).
Every hour, no matter where I would be,
I picked up the phone hoping that someone had left a message for me.
I tried to get the word out that a new dentist was in town.
I had gone to apartment buildings and businesses, spreading flyers around.
People were skeptical as they saw me coming with my stack of papers, going from place to place.
"Oh boy, what's she selling?" was written all over their faces.
I tried to be friendly and pleasant to everyone I would meet.
The first impression was as important as the words I would speak.
I also tried advertising to new residents near my location.
I paid a company to send "coupons" out saving me the frustration.
They promised a 5-7% response which was better than none.
I just hoped that I would get one!
After all, I was starting this practice from scratch.
I would take any patient they could "dispatch".

On my first day of business, I was excited in every way.
By some miracle, I had five patients on my opening day!
I hired one employee that someone had recommended highly.
Her name was Cindy, she was pleasant but she acted shyly.
She answered the phone, assisted me with patients or whatever
else had to be done.
She filled the job well although she didn't seem to be having
much fun.
Many of her days were spent doing very little.
Business was steady. It was slow but not brittle.
It was growing each day as more patients were added to our
roster.
I tried so hard to build rapport with patients so relationships
would be fostered.
It wasn't easy and got harder as the days went by.
I was still working at the dental clinic and time really did fly!

One day at the dental clinic, an assistant named Yvonne was
hired.
She was so bubbly and happy. Her enthusiasm made me tired.
But we instantly became friends and I told her about the
practice I had started.
I told her I would be leaving the clinic soon to work in my own
office full-time.
She perked up and smiled and offered to help me in the mean
time.
She said she would be happy to leave the clinic and work for me
right away. She said she would love to see me become successful
someday.
So that was how Yvonne became my first "true" dental assistant.
She seemed too good to be true; never resistant.
Always willing and able to do whatever I asked of her.
Yvonne and I became an inseparable pair as it were.
She was my right hand in the office and a trusted friend.
My patients really liked her. They didn't just "pretend".

Yvonne and I would sit around thinking of ways to attract more
patients when we weren't busy.
Sometimes I'd get so discouraged I'd become dizzy.
But Yvonne had a way of cheering me back up.
She said we'd better prepare to be old ladies still doing dental
check-ups. She said that one day I'd have so many patients I
won't know what to do.
But when you're sitting around just wishing, you wonder
whether or not it could be true.
Today, looking back on it, I can honestly say that by the grace of
God, I've never had a hopeless day! Even if it started out bad; it
ended up well.
By some miracle, I left the office feeling just swell!
Time went by very fast.
I felt settled in my office at last!
But something was missing from our lives; a void I could tell.
Something........no, SomeONE I had known so well!
Then one day a patient's husband invited me to church.
He was confident I'd enjoy his church. He believed if I came to
visit, I'd end my search.
I don't even know how he knew we were looking for a church
home.
The Lord must have put it on his heart to tell us we no longer
needed to roam.
I told my husband I wanted to visit the very next Sunday.
He agreed. We attended and it felt good in every way.
We knew immediately we had found a congregation in which to
belong that September. We visited a few more Sundays before
walking down the aisle both to rededicate our lives to Christ
and to become members.
The people in the congregation were very welcoming, shaking
our hands with a smile.
The preacher gave dynamic sermons that lasted a while.
The music was heavenly; the singers were truly blessed.
Going to church became our haven of rest.

Church felt so comfortable and familiar to me.
It was one of the fondest memories from my childhood, you see.
It was through church that I realized where all my help came from.
The Lord was there with me the whole time, and then some.
He worked overtime to make sure I didn't stray too far from the straight and narrow. Like the song says, "His eye is on the sparrow
and I know He watches me".
So everyday presented a new and different challenge or issue.
I thought that once I became a dentist, I'd no longer cry over boxes of tissues.
Expanding and hiring new staff members became a chore.
Many times I'd hire someone I thought was perfect, then had to "show her the door".
The hardest part of being a practice owner was managing the staff.
Every dentist I know just wants to practice dentistry, less the "chaff".
All dentists contend that we weren't taught how to be managers in dental school.
But when we open a practice and become the boss, we must learn how to "rule".
By God's grace, I still made it through.
Although I just had to "take it", no one really knew I didn't have a clue.

Chapter 8
My Siblings at Home

Meanwhile, back in Youngstown, grandma was having trouble
with each kid.
Milton was rebellious and hanging out in the streets, doing
whatever grandma would forbid.
It was a tough situation and they needed help badly.
I offered to help grandma but she refused it, sadly.
Andre and I were willing to take Matthew (my youngest
brother) to live with us.
But when we told her, she just kept making a fuss.
The situation kept getting worse, not better.
I would call to keep offering help and even send long letters.
Finally, the problem escalated so much that something had to be
done.
I resorted to the legal system to try to get custody of
Matthew. That's when the real problems had begun.
I never expected this matter to go this far.
Grandma seemed so unreasonable that I found it bizarre.
I retained an attorney and grandma did too.

We went back and forth to court. The family divided. It seemed too crazy to be true.
Finally the judge ordered that I take Matthew every other weekend and during his breaks from school.
I wasn't sure if that was sufficient time to make any difference but it was the judge's rule.
During the weekends he spent with us, we spoiled him rotten and he got a "pretty good deal".
We took him to the movies, shopping and game rooms and treated him to many restaurant meals.
In retrospect, I know that spoiling him was the wrong thing to do.
But at the time, that was all I knew.
Later on, I started helping him with reading.
Matt was such a poor reader so much help was he needing!
He seemed embarrassed about it. He wasn't self-assured.
He didn't want my husband to hear him struggle with words.
My heart sank as I wanted so badly to save him.
I felt I owed it to my mom even though my time was slim.
I took Matthew to be tested for a learning disability.
The test results were negative. He had the capability.
So all I could do was encourage him to try harder.
I thought he'd be motivated by my own story, but to him it didn't matter.

Meanwhile at the office things were coming along.
After a while, it seemed like each day was "the same old song".
Back in Youngstown, my sister Sophawn decided to attend dental assisting school.
She had not spoken to me about it. I thought it was odd, but still pretty cool.
Sophia and I had tried so hard to encourage her to get an education.
She insisted she just wasn't "college material" and instead wanted a vocation.

She had a hard time finding a job in Youngstown as a dental
assistant.
But she pressed on and remained persistent.
Sophawn never actually came out and asked if I would hire her
in my practice, but she did hint around to it a few times.
Only problem was, she would have to commute 1 hour to
Cleveland and back each day and she didn't have a dime.
She also had a baby girl, Kaylen to contend with. So the prob-
ability of commuting and finding a babysitter was stiff.
However, my cousin, Tammy from Youngstown applied for a job
with me.
I hired her on the spot as she promised to be on time each day
with glee.
Tammy kept asking about Sophawn working for me too.
I told her "I don't think she could commute as easily as you."
Tammy said "we can ride together and share the cost".
I replied "let's ask her if she's 'game'. Right now it's a toss".
So I called Sophawn, she agreed and everything was set.
She and Tammy began riding up to the office together in all
kinds of weather; dry or wet.

One day I panicked as I realized my only two staff members lived
so far away.
If anything ever happened to one of them, I'd be stuck by myself
that day!
I must mention here that Yvonne no longer worked with me.
My husband had finished his program and opened up his own
office, you see.
He needed someone to help him in starting his own practice just
then.

I made the sacrifice and let Yvonne go to work for him as she
was the best person for a new business.
Her great personality and flexibility were priceless; but it was
hard for me to see her depart.

However, it all worked out in the end and what kind of a wife
would I be not to help my husband in his time of need?
God always blesses us when we give from the heart.
Fortunately it was a lesson I learned right from the start.

Tammy did not stay with me that long after all.
She said she was going to start college in the Fall.
So I asked Sophawn if she'd like to move to Cleveland. She said
"yes" but that she needed to save money first.
I told her I'd give her a loan if worse comes to worse.
But we decided it was best if she moved sooner and no longer
roam.
So I loaned her the money and Cleveland became her home.
I helped her find a babysitter and soon she was all set.
She said she was grateful to me and would never forget.
That was how my sister came to work for me.
There were times when she was my only employee.
So I appreciated her. I thanked God for her and treated her
amicably.
We actually made a good team although people warned against
hiring family.

As my brother Matthew grew older, grandma really couldn't
handle it any longer. Finally she let him come to live with us
and we prayed that somehow he would grow mentally stronger.
However, by this time, he was a rebellious teen and as time
passed his rebellion grew even more.
His big brother, Milton had already gone to prison for armed
robbery of a convenience store for 3-5 years.
I wanted so badly to "save" Matthew from heading down the
same path it would bring me to tears.
He had potential although it was an awesome task.

We were ready to purchase our first home and felt we needed
"space".

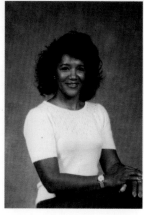

My dear mother, the late Mrs. Zelma Glenn. The most important person in my life!

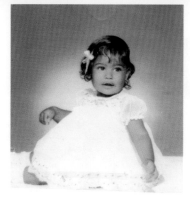

Me, 1966
18 months old

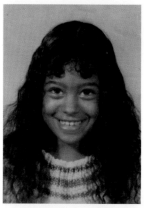

Me, Sabrina Glenn
Third grade

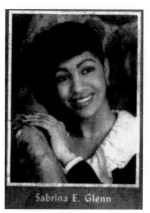

Sabrina E. Glenn

Me, Yearbook picture
Graduation from
High School 1983

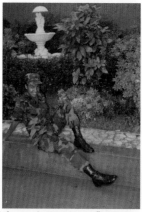

Me in Army camoflauge gear
1983, Fort Sam Houston
San Antonio, TX

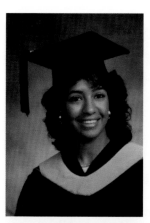

1987, Bachelor of Science,
Biology
The Ohio State University

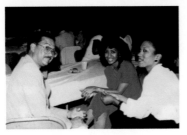

Left - Dr. James Hovell (my mentor), me, Penny Way-Wells (friend from college) at my graduation party from undergraduate studies

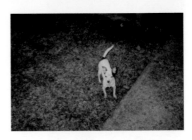

My first doggie "Chica Pica"

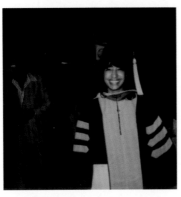

Dental school graduation 1987 Ohio State University

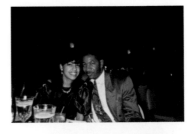

Me and my "king" André Mickel prior to our marriage

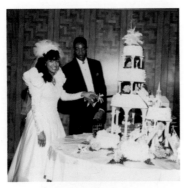

My wedding May 30, 1992 to Dr. André Mickel

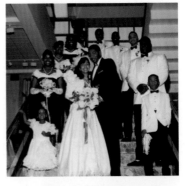

Siblings and friends in my wedding from left - Jaquela (cousin), Sophawn, Suzette, Selena, Sophia, Rudy (Andre's brother), Milton, Mario (Andre's friend), John (Andre's frend), Matthew

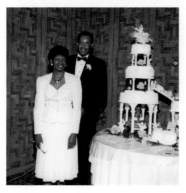

Andre's parents
Left - Late Archy D. Mickel
and Lovie A. Mickel

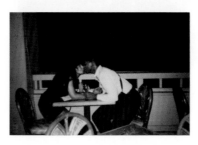

Our honeymoon

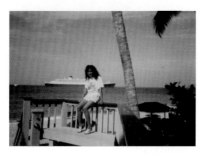

1992, St. Thomas, V.I.
Our honeymoon - the most beautiful
place I had ever seen in my life up
until that point!

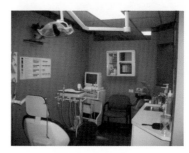

My dental office
Cleveland, Ohio

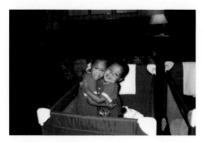

My sons
Left - André, Alexander

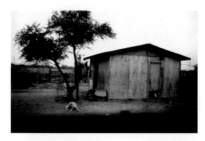

Nuevo Laredo, Mexico 1996
Our missionary trip. This is a typical
home in the areas of the people we
provided dental care for

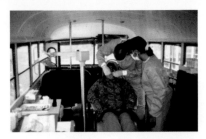

Missionary trip, 1996
André, me and a Mexican patient
on the "dental bus."

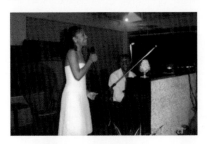

I'm singing in St. Thomas to my
husband for our 10th anniversary.

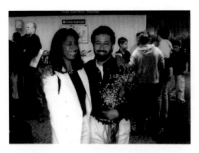

2004, Left - me, Fareed, my long
lost brother! Our first meeting at
the airport in San Francisco

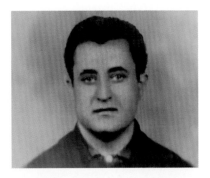

My late biological father, Ali
Hamood Hasan Algahim

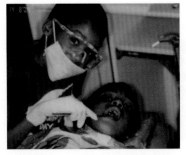

My kids - André and Alexander
Future dentists?

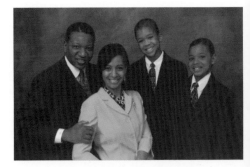

Current family photo
Left - Dr. André, Dr. Sabrina,
André, Alexander

We figured living in the "country" would be our escape from the daily "grind" and get Matthew out of the negative environment he used to face.
There's a story to our home search and home loan process.
We just weren't confident that we'd be approved. We were actually sort of stressed.
So we took it to the Lord in prayer asking for his Holy will.
It's always the best approach since God has more information than either of us ever will.
We found the "perfect" house; contemporary styling, a huge yard and neighbors afar.
The drive to work for both of us would be about 20 minutes by car.
We made an offer so close to the asking price, it couldn't be denied.
But neither of us knew in our naive minds that we were getting "fried".
In spite of it we prayed and asked God to intercede while waiting for the answer about our offer hoping it wasn't contradictory.
The answer came back so quickly; within the same day, in fact; we gave God all the glory for what we considered a major victory.
The sellers accepted our offer and threw in the refrigerator and washer/dryer set as an added bonus.
We were elated but had another hurdle to jump-the bank's decision about our creditworthiness.
Both of us had maintained an excellent credit history.
We shared the same belief that one should pay your creditors consistently
and on time. There was no mystery.
However, we were caught up in doubt hearing others tell of being denied loans because a community wants to exclude African-Americans along with some other depressing thoughts.
Andre refused to be defeated and used everything he had ever been taught.

He decided that we'd put together a unique loan application package that would at least receive extra attention if nothing else.
We put a very neat folder together and on the outside carefully placed a picture of the home we desired along with pictures of ourselves.
We included a preface on page one describing why we desired this particular home exclusively.
We included copies of our resumes and curriculum vitas along with every single document the bank required so seriously.
At the appointment with the loan officer, Andre handed her the folder and apologized for making it look like a book.
She said "O.K., but why do you think you won't be approved for the loan considering how good your credit ratings look?"
We didn't know why we had gone to such extremes but felt led by the Lord.
Perhaps we wouldn't have been approved had we not gone "overboard".
Within a week we received the good news.
We were actually approved to receive the loan we must use!
We thanked God for it as nothing should be taken for granted.
We know that God has control over the entire universe, as well as our own planet.
It was like a dream to become a home owner for the first time; especially to have such beautiful property; so peaceful and sublime.
The only nagging problem was we were so far from our church; a 45 minute drive.
Still we made it to Sunday school and morning worship every Sunday considering it a duty and necessity to survive.
We took Matthew with us to church. He needed God's word.
He wasn't too happy about it some days telling me it was absurd.
I wouldn't let him get away with it as he needed the example on which to grow.
The Bible commands us to "train up a child in the way he should go".

My husband's practice was coming along just great.
He was determined to become the best in the country, city and state.
He wanted to make getting a root canal a relaxing experience, a "piece of cake".
It seemed like an impossible task. But if anyone could do it, it was Andre K. Mickel! Make no mistake!
He succeeded in making his office delightful to all; the senses.
As you walk off the elevator, approaching his suite, the aroma was "delicious".
He outfitted his office with massaging, reclining chairs and soothing eye masks.
He made his office seem more like a spa; not an easy task.
From there
His success escalated. To God be the glory!
God had blessed us twice. We each have a divine story.

Chapter 9
Our Missionary Trip to Mexico

One day Andre received a call from "Cleveland Magazine".
They had selected him to be one of Cleveland's "50 Most
Interesting People of the Year".
They had heard about his office through the "grapevine". The
information was not volunteered.
At first I couldn't understand it. It seemed like a useless waste.
But God had a plan. He was working his amazing grace.
At a cocktail party to honor the 50 most interesting people, we
met Norm, a fellow Cleveland "celebrity".
He was being honored for his unique missionary group's ingenuity.
The group converted old school buses into mobile clinics;
medical and dental.
They focused their energies on helping all people, but helping
citizens in the poorest countries was central.
These missionaries actually drove old school buses to places like
Mexico to not only save souls for Jesus but also provide free care
for the mouth and body.

The only problem was they had no dentists to do the dentistry.
They needed somebody.
"Somebody" turned out to be Andre and me!

Shortly after the cocktail party, Andre made a "decree".
He said, "WE'VE been called by God to go to Mexico with that group.
I almost fainted as his words threw me for a loop.
But after the initial shock, I couldn't argue with him saying he was called by God, as His will we constantly seek.
We had to leave the day after Christmas to be on the road for 2 whole weeks. At first I didn't know how I would manage in the meantime. How could "I" be away from my dental office for 2 week's time?
Andre kept telling me to "let go and let God". I tried with all my might but it still felt odd.
We had to have everything arranged just right.
I told as many patients as I could about my plight.
I arranged for a "back up" dentist in case a patient had an emergency while I was away.
And Andre's parents would keep our 2 German Shepard's during our entire stay.
So everything was shaping up and I no longer had anything to worry about.
Finally, the big day came and we were full of anticipation and doubt.
Doubt surfaced when we arrived at Norm's house and saw the bus we'd be riding on for days.
It was literally an old school bus painted black, which was "spooky" in some ways.
We arrived at Norm's house at 6 a.m. the day after Christmas.
We were the first ones to arrive, shortly thereafter; the bus was full, alas.
We met our fellow missionary brothers and sisters and discovered we were the only dentists in the bunch.

The majority was going to witness and to win souls for Christ.
Some would be doing simple tasks to show Christ's love like serving our Mexican people lunch.
All would be done in the name of Jesus Christ our Lord and Savior.
We were going in His name, not seeking any man's favor.
The group was exceptionally friendly and welcomed anyone to come along and "run the race".
We started with prayer before the bus even left its parking place.
Andre and I felt very comfortable with them although they were strangers.
However, we were concerned about that old black school bus.
Was there danger?
We said our own prayer knowing that through Jesus, safely we'd be kept.
Almost as soon as the bus pulled off Andre wrapped up in a blanket on the bus floor and slept.
He seemed so peaceful and calm. I just hoped he wouldn't slide and slip.
The only overnight stop would be in Texas, 18 hours from the start of our trip!
There were 2 drivers who took turns at the wheel.
The rest of us sang, gave testimonies about what God had done for us and enjoyed a lot of meals.
Actually, the drive was not nearly as bad as we thought it would be.
We drove through snow and inclement weather but arrived safely.
The experience in Mexico was one we shall never forget; just the best!
When you help others, God makes YOU feel blessed.
You certainly learn from helping others who are less fortunate than you.
You'll also appreciate the things others don't have but that you do.

Even the little things like fresh, clean, running water to drink.
The Mexicans had to collect rain water in huge aluminum
containers. There were no sinks.
This water was used for everything from bathing, cooking and
drinking to doing the laundry.
It couldn't possibly be a situation that was very healthy.

We slept overnight in a hotel in Texas.
Each morning we drove the bus over the border praying that the
border patrol would let us.
We were there to do the work God had sent us there to do.
I was so amazed at the sights as we drove through.
Our first stop was at a church to drop off thousands of shoe
boxes full of little things we all take for granted everyday.
These boxes were Christmas gifts for the children, I should say.
Each box contained toothbrushes, toothpaste, dental floss, soap,
deodorant, shampoo, pencils, pens and paper.
The boxes were labeled for either a girl or a boy.
The girl's boxes included hair ornaments, and dolls, while the
boy's boxes contained action figures, "hot wheels" or any kind of
toy.
The boxes were distributed at a church by the congregation there.
Everyone seemed so happy just to have the opportunity. God's
love and the Holy Spirit filled the air.
Other aspects of our ministry included setting up showers on the
school buses (Norm's group had already taken and left several
other buses there already equipped for different purposes) and
giving haircuts to the boys and the men.
It felt so natural to us. Nothing else mattered, certainly not the
color of our skin.

Andre and I were accompanied by a dental hygienist and we
worked the "dental bus".
Two dentists and one hygienist to treat thousands of people;
there were only the 3 of us.

People lined up for miles to receive our free service; elderly
women and men down to the smallest kid.
We first asked if anyone had pain and some did.
We had to use the little Spanish language we knew in order to
communicate.
Andre and I took care of the people in pain first while the
hygienist cleaned teeth and gave instructions on oral hygiene as
each person would patiently wait.
The first day was extremely long and we thought we'd never get
to help them all.
But they waited patiently for us.
One elderly lady came with a swollen face so bad that a hole on
the outside of her cheek exuded pus.
After we removed the infected tooth she was so appreciative
that she returned later with a dish of food she had prepared as a
gift of gratitude.
We told her that we did it all in the name of Jesus and we
maintained a humble attitude.

The one physician who accompanied the group did not ride the
bus all the way to Mexico.
She had flown to Texas and checked into the same hotel to
meet us.
She provided vaccinations and medicine and took care of many
who were suffering and in pain.
I was reminded of Jesus, the Great Physician, and the significance
of His Crimson Stain.
Others in our group sat down with the Mexican people and
witnessed to them in Spanish about Christ and His love for
every man.
After all, to spread the Gospel was our main mission. We were
determined to do all that one group of saints can.
The gifts and services we provided were tokens of love.
Our hearts and minds were inspired from up above.

How serious is Jesus' ministry? His love and concern extends across every border.
We were called to do what Jesus would do (DWJWD- my preferred way to say this) in any order.
Our group drove to six different poverty stricken villages and did the same in each one.
We visited an orphanage to build a fence around it. Our work had just begun.
Later Andre & I discovered that the fence was being built to protect the children; to give them some relief.
Men were coming in at night, raping the little girls; it was beyond belief!
We prayed and cried and asked for God's mercy and grace.
He is a mighty way maker all we need to do is "taste (& see that the Lord is good)".
Each village was different and we had to improvise any way we could to make use of all we had come to do.
Each person we took care of was very grateful and we felt a sense of safety and well-being the entire time, too.
By serving, both Andre and I felt we were blessed as much or even more than each person we served.
The Bible tells us that "It is more blessed to give than to receive" and God had already given us much more than we deserved.
During that trip, I received a "charge" from God. I felt an overwhelming feeling to begin a family of our own.

Chapter 10
Two Baby Boys!

We were about to enter into a new role in our lives; the "parenting zone".

I had always wanted to adopt the first child. I had already told Andre this even prior to our marriage and he accepted and had no issue with it.

I recall his saying "these are the things I love about you. You're generous, humble and mild".

We decided together that we would start the adoption process once we got home.

We prayed that God would lead us in the right way so there'd be no room to "roam".

At the same time we prayed that God would take charge and that His will be done.

Meetings with counselors, social workers, attending classes and home visits were underway, the process had begun.

The classes were very meaningful to help us understand the dynamics and emotions we were about to face.

We decided we wanted a new born baby boy in any case.

We were told that statistics show girls were adopted quicker and easier than boys at any stage.
There were many more African-American boys ending up in foster homes until they were "of age".

I recall going to the very first class and meeting 3 other families going through the process as well.
Each had a different reason for being there as we would all share our tale.
One couple had suffered several miscarriages. Another couple had been unable to conceive. There was also a single woman there who wanted a baby girl, I believe.
We were shown a video tape that explained how great of a need there was for people to adopt black boys rather than girls. So it was true.
That video helped confirm for us that we were doing what God would have us do.
Following that presentation, one of the other couples changed and made a baby boy their choice.
God indeed works in mysterious ways; I began to rejoice!

During the final class, I recall feeling extremely hungry. I felt as though I couldn't wait for lunch.
This was a new experience for me; an overwhelming desire to "munch".
Since it was so strange, I sensed something was abnormal. The hunger was way too intense.
I ate so much that afternoon. I felt my hunger and thirst could not be quenched.
I asked Andre to stop by the pharmacy on the way home from the adoption class meeting.
I told him that I felt funny and needed to purchase something.
I went in alone and purchased an early pregnancy test.
When we arrived home, instead of eating more or trying to get some rest;

I immediately took the test.

To my surprise, 2 lines were present and I realized I was pregnant, in fact!

I remember telling Andre, "You are going to be a dad, Jack".

He said "Yes, whenever we get the baby. The process is not through".

My response was immediate "No, there's one growing inside of me too."

"You're pregnant?" Andre did not believe me at first. He started to walk away.

So I showed him the test results and he couldn't argue. He decided to stay.

With my eyes opened wide, I looked at him and asked "What are we going to do now?"

Andre very calmly responded, "Has our reason for adopting changed somehow?"

"Are there still other children out there who need homes in which to live?"

I could only say "yes". That fact hadn't changed just because of this new birth that God had blessed me to give.

So that was the day we discovered we would soon have two babies in our arms.

Both from God, but coming to us in different ways; we had no time to be alarmed!

Again, God works in mysterious ways.

He already had our family arranged for us. It was only a matter of days.

Once we told our adoption social worker about our situation, she immediately informed us that we should discontinue the adoption.

We told her we wanted to proceed because our reason for adopting had not changed with this addition.

She tried hard to convince us that it would be too difficult to have 2 babies so close together now.

However, we felt God charging us to press on anyhow.
The social worker, Dina, told us she was going to start "showing
us" babies and that we did not have to accept any baby we
didn't "like".
We must have given her a confused look because we'd never
met a baby we didn't like.
We told her that we would accept the first baby available to us.
Our only requirement was that he was African-American and
indeed, a boy.
God was in control of it all and even the rest.
She repeated that we still had the opportunity to choose.
She didn't understand that our charge from God was tight and
not by any means "loose".
It was March 7, 1997; Dina called us and told us that she had
our baby boy.
He was born on December 30, 1996. We were filled with joy!
The baby was 3 months old and I was 3 months pregnant; how
ironic!
It was like getting a blessing before the blessing was actually
"due". It was fantastic!
I had one on the inside being formed inside my womb and God
GAVE me my first-born at the same time. There was enough
room! (in our hearts and home).

When I first laid eyes on the baby, he was sound asleep.
I help him in my arms and he awakened without a "peep".
Then he suddenly looked up at me with a surprised face and
turned his head to look around the room for another.
It was quite obvious he was looking for a familiar face, his foster
mother.
As soon as he saw her, he cried and couldn't be comforted.
I began to feel sad knowing that even at this young age he had
to suffer yet another tremendous change.
My heart ached but it was also a sweet feeling knowing that
God had planned all of it; however strange!

We weren't able to take him home that particular day; but we were promised we could in the days ahead.

That was all part of the process of being "shown" a baby instead.
It wasn't long before he came to live with us and my heart would melt.
We named him Andre; the first born should have his father's name, we felt.
We also gave him Andre's father's middle name, therefore, Andre Delano Mickel was welcomed into our family; so sweet.
It wasn't easy but at the same time it was a special treat.

I continued to work at my office 4 days each week.
So little Andre needed a babysitter; a "nanny" we'd seek.
Once we found the right person, she came to our home each day while we went off to our offices; our daily ritual.
I cherished the other 3 days I spent with baby Andre as bonding was essential.
Both my husband and I wanted quality time with him and took him everywhere we would go.
He sat with us during our entire Sunday school class and morning worship service a lot.
It seemed that Andre was quite a smart little boy.
He wasn't content just to play with this or that new toy.
He wanted contact with a human being. He was a little "sponge".
He quickly adapted to his new routine; first order of business was breakfast and bathing to remove any "grunge".
If we decided to "put off" his breakfast he was clearly NOT a "happy camper".
As he grew older, if we waited too long to get him dressed, he'd remove his PJ's and place them in the hamper.
He began to talk early as well. Being that I was a first-time mother, I didn't really know he was so smart.

I found out later just how advanced of a child he was right from the start.

He stole the nanny's heart with his charming and loving ways.

But he had to be watched closely due to his curiosity growing each day.

It was difficult for me as my belly, my mood and my patience changed each month, day and week.

Sometimes I felt so tired and weighed down , I felt it hard to speak.

Still I didn't regret my plight in life being so busy and so trying.

I did my best to be a good mother to Andre, realizing God was responsible for our tying (together).

My nine months passed slowly as any pregnant woman will admit.

I ate like crazy and still worked hard. I was blessed that I rarely felt sick.

My husband liked to tease me and call me "cute" names like "monster".

He said I moved slow and devoured food. He was quite the "prankster".

However, he supported me in every way and cherished our special predicament; although I wasn't very kind and felt severely burdened.

Andre seemed to understand and did not become too "hardened".

He allowed me to sleep when baby Andre woke up in the middle of the night. For this I am forever grateful.

He did what was right, in spite of my sometimes acting 'hateful".

I realized that I had a great husband. He set himself apart.

He wanted to make me happy and take an active role in the family right from the start.

It was getting close to my due date and I felt as if nothing was happening. Besides the baby growing larger along with my belly

and the thought of waiting any longer, I was rejecting.
The baby didn't move much and went against all I had read
about "what to expect while I'm expecting".
I had already had the ultrasound procedure at 3 months into the
pregnancy and discovered I was carrying a boy. To be precise;
the doctor's exact words were "it's a boy and he's not bashful".
She was referring to his private part being displayed on the
screen so obvious. However we needed to be watchful.
He was also in the breeched position, meaning he was growing
right side up instead of upside down.
She reassured me that more than likely at some point during the
pregnancy before birth, he would turn around.
She was not my regular OB/GYN.
She was the radiologist who had just stepped in.
So every time I visited my regular doctor, I asked if he could tell
if the baby had turned inside my womb "bed".
He said he felt "hair" when he examined me so it had to be the
baby's head.
I accepted his explanation and trusted his judgment. I had no
reason to doubt my caring, humble doctor.
Furthermore, God was in control. He was the True Doctor!
Eventually my due date came and I had an appointment with
my doctor again. Although I wasn't blaming him, I expressed my
impatience in the nicest possible way.
He told me to try to be patient because the baby would be born
now "any day".
I was about to let him leave the room and something within me
said "speak".
As he walked out the door, I stopped him, overcoming my
quality of being so "meek".
I said "Doctor, maybe you should know that the baby seems
frantic at night. All day he is still, but while I'm asleep he moves
with all his might".
The doctor became very concerned and decided to hook up the
fetal monitor before he let me go.

This turned out to be a serious matter; something he needed to know.

He said "the baby's heart beat is irregular; you need to go to the hospital immediately."

I told him I would go later because I had to go back to the office to see patients intermittently.

He said "No, Dr. Mickel! We must save your baby!"

I then realized what I was saying sounding like a foolish lady.

I followed his order and drove straight to the hospital right then and there.

I guess I hadn't taken the fact that there was really a baby inside me seriously enough. I kind of left it "up in the air".

But here is more proof that God is in control. His will we should always seek.

Once at the hospital an ultrasound confirmed the baby was still breeched.

I couldn't imagine what would have happened had I not spoke up;

We were saved from some terrible possibilities that could develop.

The voice within me- a Divine gentle whisper to "let go and let God"!

I thank Him!

Now we were faced with what to do and were given 2 options from both the hospital staff and my doctor; both of them.

The first option, which was recommended by the hospital staff, was to call in the "man who turns babies". Did I want that for me & my son?

Of course I questioned that procedure wanting to know the specifics of how it was all done.

I assumed that it was done from the inside of my womb somehow.

To my surprise, I was told that it was instead a quick jerk and twist from the outside. Yee-Ow!

The second option was to "simply" have a C-section procedure done.

I didn't like either and my husband said we needed to pray for God's will. With God we had already WON!

We prayed and discussed the options with the doctor that day.
It was revealed to us quite clearly that the C-section was the right way.
Still, I was afraid. That meant I must undergo surgery and be cut.
It also meant I'd have to take more time off work but.........
I had to remember just who was in control. Andre reminded me to look to God as each hour went by.
I was still so afraid. I even thought the baby and I might die.
Where was my faith? I was tested but didn't completely lose it.
No matter what would happen, God's will befit.
The surgery was then scheduled for October 4, 1997. A day I'll never forget.
We had to be at the hospital by 6 a.m.
During the drive I kept praying that the hospital staff would be kind to me; all of them!
I wasn't going to be put to sleep under general anesthesia. I'd have an epidural.
That meant I'd be awake the entire time; numb only via the spinal.
I took my CD player into the operating room with me.
Andre had 2 "still" cameras and his video recorder made 3.
The Operating room staff got a little laugh realizing Andre was so happy.
My doctor asked me what I was listening to so intently.
I said "Gospel Music". He thought it was funny and laughed cheerfully.
So far everything was going fine. A sense of peace and calm was there somehow.
My doctor was ready. He had his serious face on now.
A drape was placed in front of my line of vision. I couldn't see my stomach at all.

Andre was standing to the left of me in clear view of my belly,
beyond the drape's wall.
I felt very peaceful but kept looking over at my husband's face.
I tried to judge his reactions to whatever was taking place.
He looked as if he were going to vomit. I asked him what was
going on each time I heard a new sound.
He refused to speak. He simply nodded his head and swallowed
hard, I found.
I heard the clanging of metal and the loud nauseating sound of
the suctioning of liquid.
Then all of a sudden a loud gushing sound blared through the
room.
I reached for Andre's hand and gripped it.
I felt nothing but the next sound I heard was an unfamiliar
"wailing".
I asked Andre "Is that the baby? How does he look?" My
patience failing.
Andre remained silent as the doctor's voice I heard,
"Look at that! The cord's around his neck not once, but twice,
wrapped so tight". The doctor said it was "miraculous! It was
absurd!"
Andre had already begun recording on his video camera
exclusively.
He put down the still cameras and recorded the baby's birth
curiously.
We had no idea at the time what it had all meant. But to God
be the glory for his Omnipotence.

The doctor later told us that had we tried to turn the baby, he
could have been choked to death in a matter of a minute!
Praise the Lord! Praise the Lord! Alexander was born;
my precious little baby boy; my life to adorn.
Alexander Christopher Mickel; he was given a long name.
Now I had 2 babies! NOW my life would never, ever be the
same!

I read a wise proverb that said "before you have a baby, be
prepared to have your heart outside of your body, walking
around."
I totally understand that proverb now that Alexander entered
into our world, our home, our hearts, we found.
Immediately the pediatrician whisked baby Alexander away.
At first, I thought something was wrong. I kept asking Andre
but he had nothing to say.
Then Andre left me and followed the pediatrician with the baby.
I became worried as no one told me anything. Was Alexander
deformed maybe?
The anesthesiologist was very kind and told me to relax.
She said, "Everything's fine. It's all routine" and those were the
facts.
Very soon after, I was taken into a post-surgery room to be
reunited with my husband and my new son.
He was all wrapped up in a blanket, a cap on his head, we had
WON!
I'll never forget the first time I held him in my arms.
He felt so tender, so sweet. He had suffered no harm!
He was making some kind of noise with every breath he would
take.
He was relieved and relaxed. He had been freed from the "um-
bilical snake".
Once we were taken up to a room on one of the hospital floors,
in walked Andre's parents carrying little Andre through the
door.
Little Andre was happy to see me, but didn't seem to understand
what was going on there.
We were telling him that he had a new brother but how could
he comprehend at 9 months old or even care?
He just climbed all over me in the bed, daddy snapping pictures
and videotaping it all.
Grandma and grandpa were so happy. God had finally answered
their "call".

Chapter 11
Life with Children

Now we had 2 boys only 9 months apart in age.
I would have to explain this to everyone without becoming
enraged.
Again and again people made the assumption "you two couldn't
even wait 'til you got out the hospital" was the usual remark.
They were making assumptions without knowing the facts.
I quickly got used to hearing it from strangers even while stroll-
ing the boys through the park.
Fortunately, God blessed me with a gentle spirit so it didn't
"haunt" me too much.
Andre said it didn't bother him at all. I guess that's one area
women and men differ and such.
Most of the time, I explained to people who inquired that we
adopted while I was pregnant. But that opened another assumption "door".
"Oh, that always happens! As soon as you adopt you FINALLY
get pregnant"; that remark I heard more and more.

But as you know, we had no history of difficulty conceiving.
When I tried to explain it to people, perhaps they thought I was
deceiving.
However God knows the situation and He's the only one to
Whom anyone of us must answer. He is so dear.
"He is my light and my salvation, whom shall I fear?'
(Psalm 27:1).

I'm not especially proud of the fact that I went back to work 2
weeks after the C-section.
However, my doctor said it was fine. It wasn't done entirely by
my own election.
I was curious about why my doctor hadn't detected that
Alexander was still in the breeched position.
I asked him and his response was not one you'd expect from a
physician.
I first reminded him that he said he could feel the baby's head
each time I inquired.
"Heads and butts feel the same" he conspired.
I laughed with him at such a silly remark.
Even so, I knew more than ever just Who was in control from
my heart.
It wasn't the doctor. It wasn't me. It wasn't Andre. It was none
other than God, The Almighty!

Once you have children, suddenly they become the topic of
conversation you have with everyone you know.
Instead of "How are you doing, Sabrina?"; it's "How are the
babies?" asked by patients, church members, family and even "so
& so".
I had heard other first time parents say this happens to you but
once I experienced it, I realized it was for sure. It was so true.
However, I quickly learned that your priorities change quite
drastically once you have offspring.

I love them so much. I'd walk around the house; everyday a new
song to sing.
Andre said I had become a "weirdo".
I'm sure that a great change had come over me. I even began
liking "Play dough".
I wanted to be the best mother. Andre wanted to be the best
father. We understood!
But it wasn't easy! There was no "dropping out" of parenthood.
Before having the children, we had already moved out to "the
country" as we called it.
It was so quiet. We had complete privacy and our home on 4
acres did sit.
The kids had plenty of room to ride their little tricycles, big
wheel cars and wagons.
They even had a riding car shaped like a dragon!
The nanny was excellent. She cooked for us and even did the
boy's laundry.
She taught them things like the alphabet and numbers and dealt
with their being "ornery".

With all this help, I found out where my true weakness lies.
I discovered that I have a hard time letting other people do
things I felt I should do. This wasn't very wise.
I began to "resent" the nanny for taking care of my babies in my
place.
I secretly wished I could have a double, a clone, another one of
me with every detail, even the same face.
I even recall wishing I had a magic wand so I could do anything
and everything with great speed.
These feelings were not of God. God promised in His word to
take care of my every need.
So what was the problem? I knew God could.
I wasn't casting all my cares on the Lord as I should.
But I did acquire a great deal of humility and patience as a direct
result of having each kid.

I stayed on my knees, praying for God's will, constantly asking
what He desired for me and what He would forbid.
God always answers the prayers of His saints.
One of my friends told me about a woman who was so nice it
would make me "faint".
That was when "Mimi" entered our lives. She's definitely
heaven sent.
Her home was so close to my dental office. I was able to drop off
the boys there and off to work I went.
Although this meant more work for me at home, I was much
more content.
With the nanny, I even felt uncomfortable in my own home
sometimes. What a detriment!
Andre explained that I just hadn't been used to having anyone
"serve" me in a domestic capacity.
Although I paid her for what she did, I had no peace, so I let her
go; the audacity!
I regretted it later and apologized to her but God had already
worked everything out.
He was STILL in control. I have to shout!

Andre's mom was also a great help with the boys. She sincerely
desired to help me on purpose.
But much of the time, I refused to abuse her offers; again my
weakness would surface.
I was determined to do all of the work by myself!
Why? I don't know. I guess I just like to be as busy as an "elf".

Along with my own 2 boys, I still had my brother Matt.
He wouldn't do much work at all; most of the time he just "sat".
Matthew had lived with us for a few years.
The first year he attended a boarding school and everything
seemed "cool".
This school promised to help students get better grades.
He got into trouble pretty much every day.

122

In the beginning the school overlooked it and hoped he'd change.
Then one day I got a call in the middle of the night.
Matthew had been rushed to the hospital. It was a terrible plight.
He had overdosed on some kind of tablets for coughs and colds.
My husband was out of town and the roads were covered in snow.
I had to drive alone 1 + hours at midnight to get there with 2 baby boys in tow.
Needless to say, I was extremely upset and worried during the drive.
I had flashbacks of the day I rushed home only to discover my mom had died.
And to make matters worse, now I had children of my own.
I had to wake them up, feed them, dress them and leave our cozy home.
Driving in the dark and the snow was no joke.
Furthermore I didn't know exactly how to get to the hospital; on the cell phone getting directions, I spoke.
Once we finally reached our destination, I must have looked desperate;
rushing in with 2 babies , one in each arm.
I wanted to see Matthew. I was both frantic and alarmed!
The nurses treated me kindly; realizing I had driven so far, so late, with babies in harsh weather.
They helped keep an eye on the boys while I was in the ER seeing about my brother.
As I approached his bed, I saw he was tied down to the posts somehow or another.
He was twisting and turning and yelling out unpleasant words.
I didn't know what to say or how to respond. The whole thing was absurd!
One of the nurses asked me how I could be so calm and reserved.

What she didn't know was that I was just happy he was alive so much so that my anger was conserved.

I later became angry realizing what he had done to his body.

Then I felt guilty thinking it was my fault for sending him away from the family.

I drove back home that night praying for God to help me just get through it.

I felt so overwhelmed and over burdened, I almost went into a "fit".

But God answers prayers. I called Andre's parents and they drove from Youngstown to my aid.

Meanwhile, Matt was "life- flighted" to the children's hospital in Cleveland; needing much more than a "band-aid".

My sister Sophawn and I spent the entire next day at the hospital tending to Matt.

He was in the intensive care ward. I realized it was pretty serious as I sat.

He would need mental health counseling once he recovered.

The professionals thought it was a suicide attempt, but in fact he and another boy were trying to get "high" we later discovered.

Still he was dismissed from the boarding school and I had yet another situation in which to contend.

I enrolled him in the school district in which we lived and soon his counseling would begin.

The years started going by faster once the kids were in our lives.

They were truly a joy to have around; "the apples of my eye".

Little Andre was quite remarkable as I mentioned before.

He is an extremely fast learner and quite a "character".

It amazed us how he took in everything, big and small; in his little mind he'd store.

There are many examples I could give you.

It seemed everyday was a new experience too.

Baby Andre was both devilish and sweet in his own way with this and that.

He was less than 1 year old when he quietly placed a dead spider
on my bare thigh while at the piano I sat.
I looked down and screamed at the surprise; quickly stood;
brushed myself off, and saw his reaction.
He had his "devilish" smile face on and I wondered how he
knew he'd get a rise out of me by that action.
When he was about a year older, I recall his coming into our
bedroom with his little brother. Noticing that I was still in bed,
he turned to his brother and said, "It must be Saturday 'cause
she's not up yet, come on Alexander, let's go back to bed".
Little Andre was a "take charge" child from the very start.
My husband was amazed and kept saying "Bless his little heart".
Alexander was quite different. He was sweet, but silly.
We quickly nicknamed him "Xany", but more often I had to call
him "Silly Willy".
Little Andre laughed at Xany. He would sometimes laugh
himself to tears.
Of course Alexander loved the attention and the cheers.
Xany did things like sing loudly out of tune, running around the
house singing "shake your boo, baby" all afternoon.
The actual words were "shake your groove thang" – a 1970's
song he had heard on the "Goofy movie".®
We scolded him but he laughed even more, all the while
chanting "groovy".
We all laughed thinking it harmless as he was so young.
In fact we had spoiled him and had difficulty constraining his
tongue.
Both boys were a treasure and complemented one another in
many ways.
We wanted them to be individuals as they were together and so
close every single day.
But it seemed I couldn't help myself. I even ended up dressing
them alike .
So when we were out and about the boys got a lot of attention
and the like.

Many people would stop and say "Oh, look at the twins!"
Sometimes we'd respond, other times we'd just smile and
pretend.
It was extremely overbearing to respond to everyone who
inquired.
And after a long day of walking them in the stroller, we were
tired.
Soon enough we had to start thinking about their development
and education.
On my day off from work, each Wednesday, I took them to
Kindermusik ® classes and Art classes for both learning and
recreation.
It was difficult for me to sit at home all day with the kids; so
everything I could do, I did.
Mimi, their babysitter was so sweet. I could drop them off
anytime during the day; even in a "crunch".
But my struggle within was that I wanted to be with them as
much as possible since I worked so very much.

Things with Matthew got uglier as the year went on.
He seemed to get into trouble at every turn from thereon.
I was so stressed with him in my home because of the things he
would do.
He got into fights with other kids after school and argued with
the teachers too.
Andre had predicted many years before that we would all end up
in this predicament.
The judge had denied our petition to help him while he was still
young and impressionable.
Just as Andre said, we ended up being able to take him in when
he was no longer formidable.
Matthew started to rebel even more. He started to go into
periodic "rages".
I hoped it was just another one of the many teenage "stages".

He destroyed several walls in his room by putting his fist
through them.
He carved out pieces of wood from his desk and closet. His room
I would later condemn.
He started leaving the house while we were asleep and wouldn't
return until the following day.
I couldn't handle the stress as it became too much to bear. I had
too many responsibilities; what more can I say?
I was a mother of 2 young boys so close in age they were like
twins.
I was a wife. I had a husband who needed my attention at the
very least "every now and then".
I was a business owner and a doctor with patients under my care.
I was an employer. I had employees at the office, I declare!
That was enough. I had decided that there was only so much I
could take.
Unfortunately, Matthew was the only change I could make.
The boys, my husband and the dental practice were non-nego-
tiable.
As painful as it was, I had to let my sister Sophawn take Matthew
into her home.
I thought I would go crazy as guilt took over for a while.
I prayed sincerely and God soon delivered His child.
As the Bible scripture says "after you've done all you can, stand".
I prayed for Matthew that he would find his place in this land.

Time waits for no one and soon the boys were ready to start
elementary school.
We had heard about so many different schools and so many
different tales.
We toiled over where to send them knowing they were at high
risk of going astray being African-American males.
We made the decision that first of all we needed to be closer to
our church.

We were 45 minute's drive away from it.
In order to fully participate and get our children more involved,
we needed to be closer to church from which we could all
benefit.
So we began our search for a home that would accommodate
both our need to be close to a good school and close to our
church.
We found a realtor who was very knowledgeable about the area
we were most interested in. She was wonderful aiding us in our
search!
My husband and I are the type of people who bond with almost
everyone who does a service for us.
More often than not, we end up telling them about our love for
Jesus.
They respect it whether or not they are Christian saints.
We pray for the favor of God (FOG) and he indeed responds
without constraint.
There have been so many instances in our lives where we've
been witnesses to God's divine intervention.
It cannot be explained any other way. It couldn't be any man's
invention.
The realtor "fell in love" with our family and we felt it was
sincere.
She hugged and kissed the boys at each home showing and to
her, we were endeared.
After seeing many homes in the area, finally we saw the One!
It was located 10 minutes from our church and it was within
walking distance of the school we had chosen for our sons.
It was quite a blessing and we praised God from the start.
Everything fell into place as planned; each and every part.

Moving day was quite a task; bigger than we first thought.
"2 men and a truck" were not enough, so much more help was
brought.
You don't realize how much junk you have acquired.

Becoming a "pack rat" was not a goal I had aspired.
The entire move lasted 19 hours…. non-stop.
We hadn't planned it very well. My patience went "over the top".
I couldn't blame anyone but myself for the situation we were in.
We were so tired of looking at the boxes from the very beginning until the end.
Once it was all over, we felt such relief.
I'm sure the movers felt the same as 19 hours of moving was beyond belief.
From my point of view, we were moving into a mansion now.
It was a 7 bedroom house with a pool. All I could say was "Wow"!
The fact that I had "beat the odds" so to speak,
could only be attributed to God's will, not to me, as I'm so weak.
A home is a "material thing" that many people use to "measure" success.
As God is the head of my life, that fact I must contest.
As the scripture says, "What does it profit a man to gain the whole world and lose his soul?"
Acquiring a nice home is not my ultimate goal.
I want to live forever with God and to feel the warmth and security of being His child.
I have so much to be thankful for.
The Lord God has provided more and more.
I cannot help but think about my mother although she's resting in peace now and her earthly work is done.
I had always dreamed of buying HER a big home.
Now it has all come into perspective; her heavenly crown she's won!
Our lives on earth here are temporary as Solomon* put it so plainly…..
"Man's whole duty is to fear God and obey His commandments" (Ecclesiastes 12:13).
Everything else is vanity!

It took a while to get settled into the new house and the new neighborhood.
Back in the "country" we had met all of our neighbors and felt a sense of "brotherhood".
Our new environment seemed "colder", harder to penetrate.
Everyone was so busy making a living, minding their own business at a fast rate.
It was quite obvious that we were back in the hectic city.
The change was for the better; no room for self-pity.
Even Andre and I became busier during this time.
Andre was called to travel and give lectures on time that was "mine".
The kids had to be without their daddy sometimes.
They realized he had to go, so it wasn't a crime.
The most shocking trip was his call to Beirut.
He would travel to the Middle East and be away for 2 weeks to boot!
I remember the day he left for Beirut like it was yesterday.
After hearing so many horror stories about that part of the world, I feared for his safety.
But Andre's incredible faith in God kept me secure.
He said, "God will protect me; I know this for sure."
He welcomed the opportunity to lecture abroad.
There would be professors from all over the world in his company. This was a real opportunity; not a "fraud".
So I gave him my blessing and watched him drive away bound for the airport.
His parents were there for the send-off as if it were a spectator sport.
Mom had a quiet and reserved demeanor the moment her son drove away.
I couldn't imagine what was on her mind, but I'm sure she started to pray.
Those 2 weeks were the loneliest 2 weeks of my life.

Although the boys were with me, the thought of my husband
being half way around the world "cut me like a knife".
He called occasionally to let me know he was safe and sound.
But that was no consolation, I found.
In my mind, I imagined a bomb exploding as soon as he hung up
the phone.
Where was my faith? I had no peace, even at home.
I briefly considered someone I should have known from the
Middle East- my biological dad!
I realized that the little I knew about that part of the world was
all bad.
But the thought quickly dissolved from my mind.
I just wanted Andre to return from the "bind".
Once again, God came through as a matter of fact!
Soon Andre arrived on U.S. soil, happy to be back.

Chapter 12

Losing Another Parent... Winning Another for Jesus

Shortly after Andre's visit across the world, another challenge
came our way.
Andre's dad became ill and there was only one thing left to say!
Andre felt in his heart that time was running thin.
He had tried to talk to his dad about Jesus Christ again and
again.
It seemed that dad had rejected Christ all of his life; he had
watched his family go to church and pray for years.
But whenever someone mentioned church or God to him,
personally, he would turn a "deaf ear".
Even prior to the illness, Andre felt the need to fight the enemy
and "reel his dad in".
"We wrestle not against flesh and blood, but against principalities,
powers, rulers of the darkness of this world and spiritual
wickedness in high places (Ephesians 6:12) ; NOT AGAINST
MERE MEN!

One day we all gathered at Andre's parent's home in Youngstown.

It was a Sunday afternoon. We put the boys in the car and drove
down.

Dad was going to have a biopsy the next morning at Akron
General Hospital again.

X-rays had shown tissue growing in his shoulder where bone
should have been.

We were all concerned believing it must be some form of cancer
as the doctor suggested.

The entire family gathered in one small room, making it feel
extremely congested.

Our uncle Eugene, dad's brother, started the conversation.

He told dad that we all wanted to pray for him before he entered
the operating room.

Uncle Eugene began the prayer shouting out so loud, his voice
sounding like a "boom".

We lifted dad's name up in prayer asking that God prevail to
heal his body and do whatever was His will.

He prayed for dad to have strength during this time and "peace
be still".

He prayed that mom would be strong and supportive of her
husband in his time of great need.

Then he asked God for dad's salvation. He had planted the seed.

When we said "Amen" and opened our eyes, dad's eyes were full
of tears.

Uncle Eugene told him everything was going to be all right and
he had nothing to fear.

Then Andre spoke up and asked his dad if he was ready to
receive Jesus Christ as his personal Savior.

Dad nodded his head in the midst of his tears; such a "sweet
gesture".

Dad went into that operating room the next day with a new best
friend.

Now that he had Christ on his side there was no possibility he

wouldn't win.
Either way, he now had an excellent prognosis.
Regardless of the seriousness of the diagnosis; "To live is Christ
and to die is gain" (Philippians 1:21).
For every true Christian, this scripture so dear, it remains.

Just as we thought, the diagnosis was cancer.
Mom asked, "How long does he have?" 3 months was the answer.
It was so heartbreaking to see someone deteriorate that way.
Everything seemed fine until this one day.
All of our worlds had been turned upside down.
It was hard to look at him and smile instead of frown.
Before long, dad was bedridden and mom tried so hard.
She fed him and cared for him, her patience didn't seem marred.
Eventually the time came for more help to be brought in.
Hospice sent aides to assist mom with the task now and again.
We came from Cleveland to visit when we could.
It seemed we couldn't visit as much as we should.
We had a mixture of feelings over this predicament.
I even thought I wanted to do cancer research; or some kind of
experiment.
We felt so helpless as all we could do was pray.
Dad's well-being and mom's strength was on our minds each day.

Time went by and soon we got the call we dreaded to hear.
Mom told Andre to come home as dad's last day was near.
A 48 hour "death watch" had begun; an emotional ride.
Family members were there by his side.
In one room many gathered to be there when he took his last
breath.
Everyone was so calm on the outside but inside was the "sorrow
of death".
The pastor from mom's church was there along with relatives
from near and far.

Dad had been such a kind, responsible man. He was a "silent
star".
He had never missed a day of work and was respected by his peers.
I remembered a cliché I'd heard while holding back the tears.
"Only the good die young"-maybe it was true; I feared.
We tell ourselves many things for comfort when we doubt.
However God knows why some things happen and what it's all
about.
After a while everyone gathered in one room, talking quietly
and carrying on.
Suddenly mom emerged from dad's bedside and whispered "He's
gone".
With heads bowed and eyes closed, each one uttered a silent
prayer.
Knowing that dad's earthly journey had ended; "Goodbye"
gentle man, so rare.
Mom was a pillar of strength the entire time.
I knew what loss felt like. I'd cry on the drop of a dime.
But mom only showed us strength and endurance.
Such a quality could only come from knowing Jesus Christ in
abundance.
She was most concerned about her adult children's well-being
and adjustment to this great loss.
She assumed the position as head of the family, ever looking
upward to the cross.
Life had to go on. I reflected on how much things over the years
had changed.
My entire life was drastically different; completely rearranged.
I went from Youngstown to Cleveland; from Miss Sabrina to
Doctor Sabrina; from poverty to "a girl on a mission".
But nothing was more important and more significant than
going from sinner to Christian".

I recall one family reunion in Youngstown. All of my mother's
relatives had traveled from near and far to attend.

A distant cousin came over to me. I thought he was my friend.
In a "not so nice" tone of voice, he began, "Congratulations,
Doctor. I never expected you to make it to doctor". I politely
asked "why not?" He replied, "Let's just put it this way; I know
where you came from".
I don't think that was a compliment; but perhaps envy over
what I had become.
I have never credited myself for what God has done with my
little life.
Furthermore, there are many others who have achieved far more
than me even in the midst of strife.
However, I'd like to pay a bit more tribute to my dearly departed
mother.
For without her influence, my life would be something other.
I often think about how my mom's living influence made such a
big difference for each of her seven kids.
Only the first three children actually attended and completed
college. The others did what mom would forbid.
Sophia, Selena and I had all finished high school prior to mom's
death.
Mom EXPECTED us to go to college and WE DID. She said it
with every living breath.
The 4 remaining children followed a totally different path. I
once blamed them for their predicaments.
I now consider them "victims" of having been orphaned now
living in the aftermath.

There's a lesson to be learned from seeing how this family would
unfold.
It's unlikely that a child will prosper without appropriate nur-
turing, guidance and love untold.
At one time, I resented the fact that my siblings always called
on me to help them financially.
I felt that if I could go to college and make a good living, why
couldn't they just as easily?

Now I realize God made me the new matriarch because of the gifts and talents He has given me.

My sister, Sophia, often reminds me that at least our 4 younger siblings have me to turn to in a time of need.

A scripture confirms this so well for me, "To whom much is given, much is required" (Luke 12:48).

God has given me so very much, to please Him, I'll aspire.

Chapter 13

Searching for and Finding my Biological Father's Family

I thought I'd seen it all and one day God let me know He wasn't
through.
He would continue working His amazing grace. His love is
ever true.
One day I sat in the hairstylist's chair discussing my sibling's
situations with her.
She asked if I'd ever considered finding my biological father (out
of nowhere)?
I did not recall telling her I had a "biological" father separate
from my sisters and brothers.
She said I had mentioned my Arabian heritage while discussing
why my hair was so thick and full; quite different from the
others (my sisters and brothers).
I told her that my mom said he died when I was ten years old.
I don't remember him and thinking about him left me feeling
"cold".

She responded that "since you are so admittedly different from your known siblings, why don't you find out if your father had other kids?

At first I laughed at the thought. After all my mom said she was raped. God forbid!

Tina, my stylist, pressed on, insisting that it would be a good idea for me to investigate this matter further.

I thought she was insane. I was 39 years old and already experienced enough drama!

The only thing I felt like doing was perhaps vacationing in the Bahamas.

However, once I arrived home, Tina's words still echoed in my head.

A few days went by and soon I found myself staying up late into the night; the last one going to bed.

I had begun my search for my Arabian family. I really did care!

There had to be someone still remaining; someone who shared my blood; someone; somewhere.

I sat in front of my computer, on-line hour after hour.

I didn't have much to work with; just the name of my father's store.

However, unaware, I also had God's divine power with me. He had begun to open each and every closed door.

I wanted to give up because the search threatened to consume me.

But I just couldn't stop; it had to be God's will, you see.

Finally, I sent an email, to the Youngstown Public Library.

I'm sure I sounded desperate and in a hurry.

I wrote that I wanted to find the owner of a store called Broadway Market that existed in the 1960-1970 decade.

I also explained that the owner was my biological father who I had never known. I said all I could to persuade.

I also asked for the names of any remaining relatives in the area.

I didn't actually expect a reply.

But within 24 hours, the library sent me his name, and 3 contact persons with the same last name, complete with addresses and telephone numbers. I was as high as the sky!

I was so happy. It was too good to be true.
I had already tried and paid money several times to on-line
search companies to locate public records and adoption records
too!
The library's information was free!
How silly of me!
Now that I had names and numbers, all I had to do was call.
I picked up the phone and put it down. I prayed. I cried. I wasn't
so happy after all.
I was afraid. What if they "rejected" me?
What if my "showing up" would interfere in the life of a happy
family?
I couldn't even make the first call.
I banged my head up against the wall.
Then I thought God hadn't allowed me to come this far only to
leave me.
It wasn't my fault I was born this way, see?
I prayed for courage. It was time to be nimble.
I picked up the phone, dialed the first number as I watched my
knees tremble.
No answer, then voice mail picked up the line.
What would I say? I had no guideline.
Quickly I stated my first name and telephone number and told
them that I believe I may be a relative.
I dialed the second number, got no answer, left the same mes-
sage; nothing else to give!
I couldn't bring myself to dial the third number.
The third time may have been the charm; what a bummer.
I awaited a return call. Days went by.... Waiting and waiting.
They must have figured I was crazy and ignored my call; so
devastating!

One day, not long afterwards, I felt the urge to take another turn.
I wrote a letter, explaining my entire situation and what I hoped
to learn.

I sent the same letter to the two different people I had left
messages for and included pictures of myself.
I expected that nothing would happen. Those letters would be
trashed or put up on a shelf.
But lo and behold! Yes! God is real!
He does things in his own time. He wanted me to be still.

It was Easter Sunday. I had been selected to sing a lead part in
the church choir.
It would be an early start to the day. I dare not tire.
I'd sing at both the 7am sunrise service and the 11am church
service.
So I got up early to leave and gave everyone a kiss.
I noticed a message on the answering machine that wasn't there
before.
I hadn't heard the telephone ring. Curious, I played the message
prior to heading out the door.
It was Bahia Algahmee! She was one of the two people I had
sent the letters to.
She said, "Sabrina, I got your letter." I felt the excitement in her
voice. This was all so new!
"Call me at work. I work nights and will be at this number until
7am if you wake up before then."
I called her immediately. I really wanted to know my kin.
I only had a few minutes to talk before I was due at church.
However, I had to talk to her. I had to continue my search.
I called Bahia and she was so nice. She said, "Happy Easter".
I was taken aback. She was Muslim, wasn't she?
I responded, "Happy Easter. Are you a Christian?"
She said "No, but we're on a mission."
She continued, "We were raised Muslim, but we have not
accepted the faith of Islam.
We are leaning toward Catholicism."
I said, "Who are we?"

She said, "Me, my 2 sisters and my brother." "Oh", I responded, "I see".

Bahia continued, " My brother and I got your letter and we never received a phone call or else we would have called you back right away."

I felt an extreme sense of relief upon hearing these words that day.

So I hadn't actually been rejected! They didn't hear my messages at all!

However, I did find it odd that two out of two never heard my call.

Bahia said she needed to do some more investigating to find out just who my father could be.

She thought her father was the only owner of Broadway Market as far as she could see.

She said her brother had talked about this matter the day before and had come to the conclusion that their dad was actually my biological dad!

And he was still alive! I immediately felt some emotion between glad, sad and mad!

Bahia said she was one of 4 kids her parents had.

Were they my siblings? Did we share the same dad?

Bahia said perhaps her father had lied to my mother and pretended to die.

Oh No! It began to sound like a soap opera! I wiped my eye!

She said that upon opening the letter, she looked at my pictures first.

She thought they were pictures of her oldest sister and started thinking the worst.

Maybe someone was playing a trick on her.

Then she read the letter and stood in shock as it were.

They couldn't believe it and figured I must be the sister they never knew.

Bahia said that she and her brother would be going to speak to

their father about this later that day, confidentially too.
They didn't want to hurt their mother by telling her this at all.
She said that as soon as she got more information, she'd call.
Needless to say, I went to church that day in utter disbelief.
Could this be true?
Was my father really alive and I had 4 additional siblings too?

I couldn't think about it too hard because I had to sing.
The melody was so sweet; let His praises ring!
The words to this song were, "He's not dead", meaning Jesus had risen from the dead.
With all due respect to my Savior, that song had a double meaning for me that day instead.
My Savior was not dead and perhaps my earthly biological father also was not dead!
I sang from the depth of my being for both services while thinking ahead.
I couldn't wait to talk to Bahia once again as I sang.
As soon as I returned home for the day, the telephone rang.
It was Bahia. She told me how she ended up talking to her mom about me and my story.
She first asked her mom who owned Broadway Market in its days of glory.
Her mom's reply was different than she had expected.
"Ali owned the store. He died before you were born", she reflected.
Bahia told me that once her mom told her about Ali, she felt free to tell her mom all about me.
Bahia showed her mom my picture and my letter.
Her mom remembered that Ali had a daughter named Sabrina (that's better).
Ali was their cousin so that made me their cousin as well.
Bahia received more information in which to tell.
She said Ali also had a son named Fareed.

As soon as I heard that name, I felt in my heart that he was the one.
Another chapter of my life had begun.
Fareed was the only other child that Ali had.
My mother told me I had a brother many years ago when she told me that Ali was my "real" dad.
I couldn't wait to hear all the details. Who was he? Where did he live? Was he married with children? I was as anxious as I could be!
However, as it turned out, she had no other information for me.
They hadn't kept in touch with Fareed, you see.
Then Bahia's brother, Anise called me as well. He hadn't talked to his sister that day. I could tell.
He repeated all the same things his sister had said.
He added that he had questioned his dad instead.
Anise seemed so "cool".
He seemed like someone I had known from high school.
His and his sister's words were one and the same.
Except for saying I'd never find Fareed with their last name.
Anise gave me the correct spelling and suggested I go to the internet to find my brother's address and telephone number.
I felt my heart sink upon hearing his words. He wouldn't help me any further. What a bummer!
But I wouldn't let that stop me from continuing my search.
Anise told me he believed Fareed was living in San Francisco with family but that I had to do my own research.
I kindly thanked Bahia and Anise for helping me as much as they had.
Without it, I would have had nothing to go on. Now I felt my search was iron-clad.
I spent countless hours on the web everyday.

I'd sit at my desk muttering, "Fareed, Fareed, please come my way".
I'd pray to God pleading for His aid.

I began to think Fareed didn't exist. Maybe it was a hoax. I was afraid.

I finally found an address for him but no telephone number was there.

I wrote him a letter and sent pictures; closing the envelope, I whispered a prayer.

I anxiously awaited his call, even hoping somehow he'd call me the very next day.

Of course, the letter couldn't possibly get from Ohio to California that quickly the "snail-mail" way.

Still, I was hopeful!

I scavenged through the mail each day.

Maybe he would write back to me anyway.

Two weeks, three weeks, four weeks went by.

Then I received my letter back, marked undeliverable. I began to cry.

I couldn't give up. I had already come too far.

I felt an urging inside whatever it took, I'd find my brother, however bizarre.

I used every possible resource available to me.

I found on-line reports and cross-references, his neighbors and relatives; all for a fee.

I had begun the search for my brother in the month of March. It was now May.

I had spent so much time on this matter. What else can I say?

Then, I prayed a desperate prayer that the Lord's Will be done.

I couldn't handle the stress any longer. It was too intense for anyone.

The Lord wasn't ready for me to give it up yet.

He had a plan for me. It was already set.

Late one evening, I was sitting at my computer entering search after search galore.

I came across a different web site; one I had not seen before.

It contained lists of names indicating people who shared the same address in a certain year, anytime present or past.

It listed the address and telephone number and the date the
information was verified last.
Fareed's name was there and so were many others with the same
last name.
I saw all of Fareed's old addresses but none were current; what a
shame!
However, my mind was busy at work.
I was trying very hard not to go berserk.
I paired up names and noted that Fareed had once lived with a
family that still had current information on the list.
There were also telephone numbers listed for Fareed that I had
not seen prior to this.
Quite naturally, I first tried to call him at the two numbers listed
there.
I called the first one and left a message on the voice mail with
care.
I must have sounded like an awfully desperate soul.
An uninvolved woman actually returned my call.
She just wanted to tell me I had the wrong number that time.
She said, "the call sounded so important that leaving you won-
dering would have been a crime."
I thanked her as she didn't have to do that for me.
But it did rule out my fear of thinking he didn't want to contact
me, you see.
I called and left a message at the second number. I couldn't
believe it but the same thing happened. A woman called and
said "you have the wrong number". It was so eerie.
My next move was to call the family that Fareed may have once
lived with but I felt a bit leery.
Since I kept running into dead end after dead end, I decided to
wait a few days to stretch and to bend.
What would I say without sounding suspicious?
I was afraid to call. Were these people vicious?
I took a deep breath and dialed the number fast.
Someone said "Hello". A real person at last!

The voice sounded like that of a little girl.
I asked to speak to Ibrahim, listed as head of household.
"He'll be home after three". I was told.
I said, "O.K. You are in California, correct?"
She said, "I don't know," A protective response, I suspect.
I was asking because of the difference in the time zone.
But she was right to be cautious; perhaps she was alone.
Still I felt rejected; I know it was irrational.
This whole process still had me tied in knots and so emotional.
I didn't want to call back. This was taking way too long.
I took a deep breath and vowed to be strong.
It was a Friday, May 14, 2004 to be exact.
Then I got up the nerve to call Ibrahim back.
I explained who I was and that I hoped he could help me.
"I am the sister of Fareed Algahim ", I said very quickly wanting
to cut it short.
"I have been trying to find him for months and hoped you can
help me. You may be my last resort."
Ibrahim replied, "Fareed Ali Hamood Algahim"; are you sure?
He has no brothers or sisters, maybe you need to search a little
more".
I replied to him that Fareed knows nothing about me and that I
have no idea how he will feel once he finds out.
Ibrahim's voice was suddenly filled with excitement.
He told me he had to go physically find Fareed . He took down
my name and number(s) and promised to call me back.
You can imagine the anticipation I had that entire day.
I was on "pins and needles", jumping every time the phone rang.
No call came that day but I was still hopeful, in fact.
The next morning was Saturday and I would call back.
I'm an early riser but decided to wait until a reasonable hour.
Had I called the west coast at 6 AM EST, I would have surely
been a bother.
So at noon I dialed the "magic" number feeling more confident
this time.

Ibrahim answered happily and informed me that he had located Fareed and would be delivering the news that same day. Again, I patiently awaited a telephone call from California, I should say.

That night my husband and I attended a formal event for the University at an elegant hotel downtown. Everything was beautiful including the centerpieces on the table. Although we had the opportunity to fellowship and reminisce with old friends from dental school, my mind was not stable. All I could think about was the call I expected from my long-awaited brother. I sat at the table smiling and holding my cell phone in my lap using my shawl as a cover. Suddenly, in the midst of our sit-down dinner, my phone vibrated on. Instinctively, I got up from my seat. Andre grabbed my arm and asked me what was wrong. I remained in motion responding, "this is my call"! "What call?", he asked as my heart raced. I yelled out, "MY CALL!", as I rushed away to find a more quiet place. In all my rushing, my handbag dropped open. I was trying to be discreet but I dare not miss the call. I answered and immediately said "hold please" as I bent down to pick up the items that would have to fall. I imagined myself as Cinderella rushing out of the ball; trying to "beat the clock" so everyone would not see me "lose it all". But during those few moments, nothing else mattered to me. Whatever those other people thought or saw, so let it be. Putting the phone back to my ear, my first words were, "thanks for holding". The noise level in the room was still so great; the conversation was difficult unfolding. I managed to hear "Sabrina?" My immediate response was "Fareed, is this really you?"

"No, this is Ibrahim, Sabrina. I spoke to Fareed today and gave
him your number. He's going to call you tomorrow." In my mind
I thought, could this be true?
I was so excited even though I'd have to wait another day to
speak to my "new" brother.
Smiling, I returned to my seat next to Andre and whispered "I'll
tell you later one way or another".
As the evening came to a close, my mind was a "million miles"
away anticipating that long-awaited phone call.
I got a little concerned thinking about the next day being
Sunday because I would be in church for a great part of the day.
I didn't want to miss Fareed's call for any reason at all. I had
given Ibrahim my cell phone number as well as the numbers to
my home and office.
So Sunday morning I didn't sit in my usual church pew 3 rows
from the pulpit, instead I sat in the back with my phone set on
to vibrate the softest.
As people passed by me, they inquired why I wasn't in my usual
spot. Since I sat in the front so often, something was odd;
anyone could tell.
I just nodded and smiled at each church member assuring them
that all was well.
I was barely able to concentrate on the church service as I held
the cell phone tightly hoping he'd call anytime other than
during prayer or the sermon.
The entire service passed without a call. I felt both a sense of
relief and a sense of disappointment. Every emotion you can
imagine, I felt them all.
I kept reminding myself that he lived in the Pacific Time Zone;
3 hours behind us.
I tried everything not to get too discouraged. Over and over I
whispered in my mind "He's going to call….he must".
Church service had ended and no call came through.
I tried to put it out of my mind so I wouldn't feel so blue.

Chapter 14

Fareed Ali Hamood Algahim

On the way home from church my mind shifted to more real day
to day stuff.
I had to get dinner ready for my family, spend time with the
kids. I already had enough.
But God is good all the time! No sooner than I walked in the
door to my house did the telephone ring showing a California
call on the caller I.D.
Instantly, a great sweat came over me and my heart started to
beat mightily.
I picked up the phone and sheepishly answered "Hello". The
voice on the other end sounded just as "sheepish". "This is
Fareed", he said in a quiet, questioning tone.
I didn't know what to say. "Hi Fareed. How are you?" Apparently neither did he because there was an uncomfortable silence
on the other end of the phone.
I got up the nerve to say, "You are probably wondering what
this is all about." He responded with a simple, "Yes". Sweat
poured from my body heavily again.

I figured he must have thought I was a lunatic or something just then.

I tried to tell my story. I asked if he was born in Youngstown, Ohio. He said, "Yes" but remained quiet. I continued, "My father was Ali Hamood Hasan Algahim. He owned Broadway Market in Youngstown and died in 1975."

Fareed with unexpected excitement said, "515 Broadway"! "Yes, I replied."

Was he going to say anything else at all?

I was prepared to be cursed and stall.

Instead the next words from his mouth were "I thought this was a dream. I cannot believe it. My mother told me I had a sister when I was 10 years old but she wouldn't say anything else about it and I dared not ask".

He spoke with a foreign accent so understanding him was a slightly difficult task.

I noticed right away that he had a humble and "sweet" demeanor. He said, "Please excuse my words as English is my second language". I didn't understand why that was the case since he was born in Ohio, but decided not to get the facts just yet.

I explained how I had written a long letter including pictures and it was returned as "undeliverable".

I also explained how I had spent 4 months searching for him and thought I'd never find him which made me feel miserable.

I asked him for a current address so I could still send the letter and pictures. I felt way too nervous to keep up this conversation.

I told him how I had planned for him to receive the letter before we talked on the telephone to deliver this "revelation".

I spoke of how I wanted to give up so many times but I truly felt led by God. He perked up at my saying "God". He asked what religion I practiced. I told him that I was a "born-again Christian". He said, "I'm Muslim".

Of course I knew this since our cousins in Youngstown already told me; the ones who helped me find him.

Then Fareed proceeded to begin this whole conversation defending the Muslim way. "It's not what you hear on television. We don't encourage violence. They have made us into terrorists. I know you hear it everyday."

I reassured him that I was not judging him for his belief in the Muslim way. I was just so happy to actually be talking to my Arab brother that day!

Then the most unusual thing happened. Fareed began to sound as if he were crying and asked "why did you wait so long?" I told him it was not by choice.

He was so sweet. I felt tenderness, genuineness and warmth exuding from his voice.

He actually WANTED to know me! Again, I had not expected that!

He reflected briefly on how he felt when he first received the news about me.

When Ibrahim told him that his sister called he thought it was a trick, you see.

I also discovered that Ibrahim himself thought I was playing some kind of trick as well since he didn't know that Fareed was born in Youngstown. Yemen was their home country so he thought Fareed was born in that far away (to me) hometown. When Ibrahim told Fareed that I had mentioned Youngstown was his birthplace, Fareed knew there was actually something to all this.

He and his mom had left Youngstown in 1975 when our dad passed away. Fareed was just 5 years old then.

Fareed told me how he cried and cried after hanging up the phone with Ibrahim and reflected on the news.

His memory was sparked and that was when he remembered his mom had told him he had a sister, making this news true!

He said he picked up the phone to dial my number and wept so much that he had to hang up before finishing the dialing.

He could not control the intense emotions that suddenly overcame him: one moment crying, the next moment smiling.

This went on for hours while I sat and waited for his call in
church that Sunday.
Then I understood why he had started out being so quiet when
we finally talked that day.
I still did not know what to say.
I wanted to meet him as soon as possible but San Francisco was
so very far away.
However, from the moment we talked, I felt an intense love for
him.
I felt in my heart that something had finally been completed but
that something else was about to begin.
I also felt that I had already achieved success in life and with
Christ Jesus, I had NEW LIFE!
And had I never found my brother, everything would have still
been all right.
But there was a lingering "unknown". Who was my biological
father? What kind of a lifestyle did he live?
What really happened with he and my mother that made me
live?
What qualities of his had I inherited? When I saw Arab people,
I wondered if they were related to me.
When I heard people speak negatively of Arabs, I felt a bit
insulted, can you agree?
I didn't know anything except that my mother was African-
American and my biological father was Arabian.
I asked Fareed questions about our father, but he could not
answer most of them.
Since he was only five years old when we lost our father, he
remembered nothing at all.
He said he only remembered seeing a picture of him in the
casket, not a great memory to have to recall.
Before ending the conversation, I told my brother I would help
him with anything he might need.
Again, so humble and kind, he graciously repeated "Thank you"
several times as if I had already done some good deed.

During the first conversation, he mentioned he had 5 kids and a wife.

The problem was his family lived in Yemen but he had to live and work in San Francisco so far from them for much of his life.

He had been an airplane mechanic but after the infamous "911" he and many others were handed "pink slips".

Since then he has been working in different fields and is content just earning a living. But the entire situation had him doing flips.

I had indeed found my "lost" brother! He was 34 years old and I was 39! But, Oh, what joy divine!

All the years we missed together.............. How would we ever make up for all that lost time?

But it was God's plan so all I can say is "Oh, what peace sublime".

God really is good all the time. His unlimited power reaches well beyond the human eye.

"I love the Lord. He heard my cry"!

Even though I knew it was, in fact, He who put the search for Fareed in my heart.

So I must believe God had given me the task right from the start.

Before ending that first conversation, Fareed told me he'd call me everyday.

I didn't think it was necessary because I wanted to actually SEE him just once face to face....somehow..... someway.

But I laughed and thought it was merely a sweet thing for him to say.

Immediately after that first conversation, I went to work on the internet and searched all day.

I had to find a hotel and airline tickets to San Francisco for Memorial Day weekend; just 2 weeks away.

Fareed could not believe I was going to fly there so soon. He must not have realized how anxious I was.

He did not realize how all my life I had a deep longing to find
out something about my biological father; just because?
All the years of wondering and fantasizing would finally come to
an end.
Now I would experience a bit about my "lost" biological half;
truly a Godsend.
I knew plenty about the African-American part of me.
I lived it everyday of my life; deeply involved in the culture of
my displaced African ancestors, you see.
Yet, just knowing that my body contained DNA from some
distant land had me yearning for some knowledge of it.
I ran into the kitchen where my husband and children were all
ready for dinner and ready to sit.
"I talked to Fareed and we're going to go meet him in two
weeks, Boo!"
I announced with glee!
Andre was happy for me and had no issue with my making all
the necessary arrangements for our last-minute trip to California
indeed.
I must have called over 50 relatives and friends. Among them
were my grandma, and all my sisters. I called my aunts in Geor-
gia, my best friend and countless others.

Memorial Day weekend couldn't come soon enough so I could
finally meet my brother.
In the meantime I prayed that our first meeting would be
beautiful and like a fantasy.
I had no pictures of Fareed but he had 3 of me.
He had received my letter within a few days of that first
conversation so at least he knew what I looked like.
He told me he waited 5 hours at the post office anticipating my
express letter!
When I heard this, I simply could not believe it, but it made me
feel so much better!
Was he really as excited about this as a little boy?

When I thought of how long I procrastinated about the search, I
felt I had cheated him out of years of joy.
He had called me after receiving the pictures. By the way, he did
indeed call everyday and was never a bother.
Happily, he said "You have the flesh of my father…. I mean Our
father".
Since I had never heard that kind of a description before, I
asked him what he meant. He said, "Excuse my English again. I
may be using the wrong words".
I asked, "do I look like our father?" He said, "Yes, very much, it's
absolutely absurd!"
When the day came to go to San Francisco, I was both nervous
and full of joy; just a mess, you see.
I was so excited I didn't know what to do and Andre didn't
know what to do with me.
The flight seemed so long because of the anticipation although
we had a direct flight from home.
I was actually going to meet my "flesh and blood" brother for
the first time! My mind began to roam!
The closer we got to landing, the more nervous I felt. My mouth
was extremely dry and my hands were wet with sweat.
What did he look like? How tall was he? A million thoughts and
visions would flash through my mind until we actually met.
I used my cell phone to call him and let him know we had
landed and would meet at baggage claim.
He said "I will be right there, Sabrina." I loved the way he said
my name.
Andre and I walked to the baggage claim area and looked
around.
But Fareed had to find me since I didn't know his face, perhaps
I'd know his sound?

All of a sudden 3 young men appeared, one was capturing
everything on a camcorder, one was just smiling and the other
was carrying a bouquet of red roses with the biggest smile and

eyes that sparkled like none I had ever seen before.
We immediately embraced as we both felt such unspeakable joy.
What a wonderful day!
Fareed kept repeating "Finally!" I kept repeating, "I am beside
myself and don't know what to say".
Fareed embraced Andre as well and then embraced me again
and again with tear filled eyes.
It was an experience of a life-time; a great surprise!
Immediately, everyone present saw the resemblance between us
two.
We are the same height, we have the same eyes, and the same
mannerisms to boot.
Fareed was accompanied by two cousins who both seemed as
happy as could be.
They were excited for us and said this situation was "like a
movie on TV".
We spent that entire weekend talking; staying up late and
waking up early just to talk.
Andre and I stayed at a hotel. Fareed lived close enough to drive
to the hotel within a few minutes. Both mornings just he and I
went for early morning walks.
He brought me coffee and donuts. He made sure Andre had
breakfast too.
He even brought food to the hotel for later after we settled in
for the night; it's true!
His thoughtfulness and hospitality was totally unexpected; a
true delight.
He took us on a grand tour of the Bay area and to meet relatives
who lived in Oakland, It all felt so right.
He did speak a bit about his Islamic beliefs, but Andre and I just
listened to what he had to say.
He was very "religious" and would leave us at the designated
times to go to the mosque to pray five times a day.
Quite naturally that weekend passed by too fast.
I wasn't totally satisfied but at least I had met my brother at last!

We headed back to Cleveland. Life had to go on.
Little did I know that my feelings for my brother would deepen
to a point of no return?
Fareed and I continued to talk on the phone every single day.
Regarding one another, there was so much yet to learn.
Our conversations revolved mostly around our different religious
practices and beliefs.
I "gingerly" told Fareed about my Christian faith, however
uncomfortable. Changing the subject was a relief.
I told him that the basis of my salvation rests on accepting Jesus
Christ as Savior and Lord.
He promptly informed me that my belief was absolutely absurd.
He stated that Jesus Christ was just one of many prophets and
that Christians elevate him to much too high a level.
I listened but at the same time I asked Jesus to hold back the
devil.
I wouldn't listen to what I considered blasphemy in the least.
This was my brother and I couldn't accept it from him in peace.

I found myself longing to go back to San Francisco to spend
more time with Fareed.
I planned a trip for the Fourth of July weekend. I felt such a
great need.
I asked my closest sister, Sophia to accompany me.
She happily agreed stating that she was just as curious to know
about the "other" half of my biological family. Fareed was one
she wanted to see.
Fareed could not believe that I was flying there again so soon;
thinking perhaps I'd be making one trip after another.
I reassured him that everything was fine and with my busy
schedule I had to take advantage of every extended weekend to
get to know my "new" brother.
I was so excited for Sophia to meet Fareed.
I wanted her to be a part of this unique experience indeed.

Sophia flew to Cleveland and we planned to fly out to San Francisco together.

When the weekend arrived, I was overjoyed; feeling as light as a feather.

I had the opportunity to get away, spend time alone with my sister; and at the same time, I'd visit Fareed, the one I longed to know.

This made me the happiest woman in the entire world; or at least I thought so!

Sophia and I would be leaving at 9:30 AM EST and arriving in San Francisco at 11:15 AM PST. We had a direct flight. However, I messed it all up. I was out of sorts.

I awakened at my usual "5:30ish" and had plenty of time to be ready to arrive on time at the airport.

I also made sure that Sophia was up and getting ready by 6:30 and intended to leave the house by 7:15 for the 20 minute drive to the airport, thus arriving at least 1 hour prior to the takeoff of our DIRECT FLIGHT.

I cannot explain what happened except that I wasted too much time fiddling around. I kept adding and subtracting things from my luggage. The luggage and I were actually involved in a fight".

I wanted to have small love gifts for everyone I had met on the first trip; all of the cousins and their children and of course, Fareed.

I bought a Bible especially for him; hoping I would be planting a seed.

By the time we headed out the door it was already 8:45. Somehow I thought we would still make it in time.

Instead, once we arrived at the check-in counter, the airline agent said "Sorry, you are too late to check in baggage and make that flight.

I was a total mess, devastated; acting so crazy I could have been placed under arrest.

I begged and pleaded with her in a way that was totally uncharacteristic of me.

Sophia promptly told me to snap out of it, stop the embarrassment and let the lady free.

The agent informed us that she could make a new itinerary and we would arrive in San Francisco by 5:30 PST after a connection in Denver.

But what a bummer! We would spend the entire day traveling and missing a precious, beautiful day of summer.

The time I planned to spend with Fareed would be decreased drastically and worst yet, I had to call him and explain how in the world I had caused us to miss our flight.

He was not at all happy when I relayed the news informing him of our plight.

He kept asking what happened as he already knew I was an early riser.

I apologized over and over not knowing what to say. I felt I had failed him somehow. He reassured me that everything was fine; he couldn't have been any nicer.

And I came to realize that he was far more interested in my safety than whether or not I had made that particular flight.

I explained to him that we had to change planes in Denver. He told me to be careful and to call him whenever I had the chance to inform him of our traveling progress, however slight.

Once we finally arrived in San Francisco, Fareed was right there waiting for us.

He told me he had been waiting for a while, anxious but calm, not making a fuss.

Sophia spotted him first, recognizing him from the pictures I had shown her and the zeal with which he was approaching us.

I dropped everything and ran to embrace him. I knew he'd be there. I had total trust.

He had rented a car for the weekend to transport us from place to place.

I was just satisfied being able to once again see his loving face.
Sophia was a great help as she is my loving sister and acted as my aide.
She tried to "school" me on the Arabic culture and religion; the little she knew; but what a difference it made.
Sophia had spent a year's tour of military duty in Kuwait (she is a Colonel in the Army Reserve) just 6 months prior to this meeting.
So she had some idea about the culture, especially a bit about the customs and the greetings.
During that visit we spent a considerable amount of time with the cousins and I really felt as if we were one big family group.
The children were delightful, happy and pleasant; as if they were doing flips and jumping through hoops.
The men were respectful and seemed to treat me and Sophia in a very special way.
The best time we spent was sitting on the backyard lawn enjoy-ing a picnic dinner on a beautiful, sunny day.
It bothered me that the Muslim ladies did not sit down to eat with us.
Sophia, the men and I sat on a blanket enjoying a great home-made meal and interesting conversation.
Perhaps the women did not sit because they spoke no English.
Regardless of the reason, they were clearly not a part of the recreation.
However the ladies presented us with beautiful gifts.
Sophia and I received a traditional dress and a very nice ring.
This undeserved gesture gave us a lift.
The women wanted so badly to talk to us for just a while.
However, I didn't speak Arabic and they didn't speak English; all we had was the universal language......A SMILE!
I asked Fareed to translate so we could converse.
He declined saying it wouldn't be proper for a man to translate for two women. Was it a curse?

So Shaima (our 12 year old cousin) tried to do the translating,
you see.
It was my first cousin named Salwa who wanted to ask questions
of me.
Salwa asked through her daughter, Shaima whether or not I
expected to have more kids.
I told her "No, two is plenty". This statement "tickled her ribs".
She laughed at first and then most curiously wanted to know
why I felt this way.
I tried to explain that my career and my two boys already made
for many a hectic day.
Our cultures were worlds apart as her full-time job was home,
family and spouse.
I wanted to address this but dared not and remained as quiet as a
mouse.
I wanted to ask if she had the opportunity to work outside the
home but I already knew the answer was "no".
Fareed had already told me that a woman would need her
husband's approval to go to college or to work.
The general rule was to keep your wife hidden from the public
to avoid the temptation of other men; as if every man were a
jerk.
I didn't question anything although I was curious about many
differences; things I had never thought of before.
It appeared that the men were all free to do whatever they
chose. Women were not. I wondered if the women longed for
more.

Once we left the relative's home, Fareed and I became extremely tired since we had been awake so early that morning
spending time sitting by the beach, simply talking.
The time passed quickly as we conversed watching other people
on the beach simply walking.
On the other hand, Sophia still had plenty of energy and

wanted to enjoy the remainder of the day; maybe even catch a glimpse of a night time star.

Our cousin, Mohamed, was driving as Fareed and I were falling asleep in the back seat of the car.

Mohamed and Sophia must have felt sorry for us two; tired and weary from both getting up so early and the overwhelming excitement of our newfound siblinghood.

Mohamed dropped Fareed off at his apartment and me at the hotel room for our own good.

Fareed and I agreed to get up early the following morning and once again spend time talking and enjoying the beautiful San Francisco sunrise.

Meanwhile, Sophia got a grand tour of San Francisco by Mohamed to my delight and surprise.

We felt very comfortable with them although they were really "strangers".

Somehow I had no doubt that Mohamed would protect Sophia and keep her from any danger.

The two of them saw fireworks and walked along the pier as it was Sophia's first time in that city.

I was so appreciative of Mohamed's hospitality toward my sister right down to his personality; as he is so very witty.

When she returned to the hotel room, she told me what a wonderful time they had.

I was so happy to see Sophia feeling comfortable and accepted just as I was accepted.

She enjoyed herself and had no concerns of being rejected.

The truth about me and Fareed is hard to swallow.

A brother and sister meeting for the very first time in 34 years is something we both consider to be God's miracle.

Our love for one another runs deep; not at all shallow.

We constantly talk about how hard it is to understand and how our love seems to grow stronger as each day goes by.

We keep asking one another the same question…"Why?"
Our discussions began to revolve around religious beliefs as we
strive to know God's Will.
Each conversation becomes more comfortable as we try to
understand the reasons for the way we both feel.
I pray that Fareed will embrace Christianity one day and he
prays that I will turn to Islam in some kind of way.
It seems like a losing battle as we are both so devoted to our own
individual faith.
But just as I told him, I have already claimed him and we will
one day share in the victory.
All of the doubt he has will be gone. It will be history!

Chapter 15

Conclusion.....It's All in God's Hands

So now here we are at the present day.
I'm the oldest of 8 now and feel responsible for them all in a
way.
You may be wondering what has become of my other siblings for
my story would not be complete without an update.
I still believe the 4 youngest are victims of a lack of proper
parenting; ultimately leading to their fate.

Sophia is a born-again Christian and we talk most everyday
although she lives in Florida, many miles away. She has her
Ph.D. and she is married. My sister, Selena lives the "single life"
in Chicago. I call her the "wild child" and pray that the Lord
will just keep her alive. She is a Radiology Technician and has a
very flexible work schedule by choice. She frequently travels
worldwide.
But I know that our God is waiting for her. He's still on her
side.
I pray that she will turn back to Him as it is only by His grace

and mercy that we are all still here.
God has given her a chance to accept Him as Savior and Lord
because He loves her so dear.
My sister, Sophawn is married and the mother of three little
girls. She works in my office and she's a beautiful singer. She's
trying to make her way in this world. I'm happy to report that
she is active in her church and trying to raise her girls to follow
the Lord.
My sister, Suzette is married with four children, 2 girls and 2
boys. She also is trying very hard to get her life together as it's a
combination of both pain and joy.
She is also committed to rearing her children "in the way they
should go".
Of course it's not easy for her but she's determined to make them
solidly grow.
My brother, Milton has been imprisoned twice.
I never know what's next with him, It's like tossing dice.
These days he seems more concerned about living "right".
He now has a 3 year old son. I suppose he doesn't want his son
to end up facing the same plight.
He lives in our childhood home watching it fall apart around
him.
He has developed a closer relationship with our father, Glenn.
They work odd jobs together through temporary services every
now and then.
Matthew lives there too and I do what I can to help them both.
Matthew's mental disorder has not improved much at all.
Worst yet, they don't always have a telephone in the house so I
cannot call.
Whenever they call me, it's usually a request for money.
Sometimes the requests are serious, sometimes funny.
Again, I can only pray for all of them and their children and do
what I can to help when asked.
Sitting back and watching people you love "waste away" is a
heart-wrenching task.

On a happier note, Fareed and I continue to talk or text message one another almost every day.

We have had some light-hearted conversations about his family in Yemen and what his children say.

He constantly tells me how his kids are so excited about having an "auntie Sabrina" in America.

They say my name over and over but speak little to no English.

I cannot wait to meet them all: Ibtihal, my sister-in-law; Mohammad and Ali, my nephews and Maryim, Negwa and Diana, my nieces.

It may be years before we actually get the chance and they are just as excited or maybe even more so from what Fareed tells me.

Only the three youngest children have passports and who knows when or if I will ever visit Yemen.

I long to meet them.

I long to embrace them.

I long to feel like family.

But for now, I must remained focused on my priorities although I've just had an experience that has changed my life.

I pray that the Lord will help me daily to stay on point like the tip of a knife.

My Lord shall always be the Head of my life. He's the foundation on which everything else is built.

Next, my husband and my two boys take priority and for this I have no guilt.

Next in line is my extended family, sisters, brothers and close friends of which now Fareed is a member.

My career as a dentist to care for my patients, make a living and give back to the community; from whence I came, I shall always remember.

The organizations I belong to are all for a good cause.

I am convicted not to waste this precious time on earth but still take some leisure time to pause.

God has been so good to me even when I virtually ignored Him.
He still keeps His promises and has filled my cup to the rim.
Trials and tribulations still lay wait for me and everyone who lives on this earth.
But to God be the glory for giving us all a second chance through Christ; His plan for magnificent rebirth!

The End

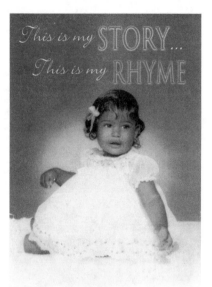

DR. SABRINA EILEEN MICKEL

To order additional copies, go to my website
shiningangelpublishing.com

Or write to us
Shining Angel Publishing
3461 Warrensville Center Road, Suite 301
Shaker Heights, OH 44122

Phone Orders 802-297-3771
Fax Orders 802-297-3326

Visa, Mastercard, Discover, American Express, Money
Order by mail. No personal checks.

Price of additional copies $19.99 plus $4.50 S/H.
(Ohio Sales Tax 7.5% and price subject to change. Call for current price)